The New Fitness Formula of the 90's

The New Fitness Formula of the 90's

A compilation of 12 points of view written by the nation's top health writers and fitness authorities

Published by
The National Exercise For Life Institute

Dedicated to collecting and disseminating information concerning the benefits of exercise, in order to convince more Americans to undertake and maintain a personal program of regular exercise.

The National Exercise for Life Institute
Box 2000
Excelsior, MN 55331

Library of Congress Catalog Card Number: 90-62773

ISBN 0-9627708-0-9

Printed in the United States of America

Notice

The information and ideas in this book are for educational purposes and are not intended as prescriptive advice. Consult your physician before starting any exercise or weight loss program.

Illustrations: Jay Colt Weesner   *Layout: Kristine Hennebry*
Cover Art: Michelle Crawford

*This book is dedicated to the contributing
writers in acknowledgment of their
continued commitment to improving
health and quality of life.*

Table of Contents

Foreword

No question about it, exercise is good for you. There exist millions of pages and miles of video footage documenting that fact over and over and over again. Researchers, including those at The National Exercise For Life Institute, have spent thousands of people years and millions of dollars proving just that fact. The problem is, we still don't exercise.

We have good intentions. At one time or another, nearly everyone has tried some type of exercise. In fact most of us have tried several...jogging, health clubs, indoor bikes....Each of which we do just long enough to lose some weight, get to feeling pretty good, and hear some compliments from the spouse. Then plop, back to the pretzels, the tube and the double buttock chair.

The whole exercise movement has become somewhat Darwinian as a result. (Take a look at the skeletons of extinct exercise equipment buried in your garage if you doubt its existence.) Though still overweight, we have learned a great deal from this evolutionary process. We know, for example, that exercise can be fun, that it doesn't have to hurt, that we can get it in lots of different ways, and that it provides a wide, wide variety of health benefits. But still we don't exercise. Obviously, there's a missing link.

Most of the exercises most people perform are aerobic exercises: exercises that enhance cardiovascular endurance, reduce body fat, increase energy, minimize stress...you know the story. It's the kind of exercise you get from your thrice-weekly workout aboard your NordicTrack or your morning run through the park. However, superb device that your NordicTrack is, scenic as your running path may be, both NordicTracking and running are *aerobic* exercises. Which means they burn fat and increase cardiovascular endurance. But they don't increase muscle strength...the missing link.

Consider for a moment the true goals of exercise. Are they really a lower cholesterol profile, lower blood pressure and less body fat? No. The true goal of exercise is much broader: quality of life. The true goal of exercise is a body that will serve you well in not just the acts of day-to-day living, but in the acts of day-to-day dreaming. In other words, the true goal of exercise is to create and maintain a body that will let you live the life you'd love to live. And that takes muscle strength.

According to James Garrick, M.D., director of San Francisco's Center for Sports Medicine and author of *Be Your Own Personal Trainer*, "There's a lot more to enhanced fitness than improved cardiovascular function. That's the one everyone talks about, but there's more to life. It doesn't do much good to be able to run across the concourse of the airport to catch a plane if your shoulder hurts for two weeks afterward from carrying your carry-on bag."

Strength training is the kind of exercise people do with barbells (no, not dumb bells), calisthenics and any of a wide variety of resistance devices. In the past, strength training has been a young man's recreation and its image has suffered as a result. That's unfortunate because a large volume of research now indicates that it should be a component of every fitness program, including yours.

Strength training provides a broad range of positive adaptations in terms of both function and health. Among those positive adaptations are increased muscle strength and bone mass, improved body composition, more energy, better posture, decreased risk of injury, and greater self-confidence and self-esteem. Some studies have even documented cardiovascular responses that include lower blood pressure and resting heart rate.

Steven Fleck, Ph.D., a sports physiologist with the U.S. Olympic Committee says, "Strength training is no longer the exclusive domain of elite athletes. Rather, the potential health and quality of life benefits will be the focus of all comprehensive fitness programs of the future."

In their new guidelines released in April 1990, the American College of Sports Medicine underscored the importance of muscle strength by revising their 1978 position stand, "The Recommended Quantity and Quality of Exercise for Developing and Maintaining Fitness in Healthy Adults," to include "strength training of moderate intensity at a minimum of two times per week," in addition to regular aerobic exercise.

This combination of aerobic exercise with strength training is referred to as "balanced fitness." Its importance as a concept has broad implications for us as individuals and as a society. It will make us healthier, more attractive, and increase both our self-esteem and self-confidence. It will reduce disease and medical costs, increase our productivity, and keep us independent for years longer. And perhaps most importantly, it will make us better exercisers because the benefits it provides cannot be denied and once discovered, cannot be ignored.

This book is a compilation of articles on the subject of balanced fitness by some of the world's leading authorities. The emphasis is on strength training simply because its importance has only recently been discovered. Explore this book. Read it in bits. Savor it. And enjoy your first step in making balanced fitness a part of you life.

Diane DeMarco
Executive Director
The National Exercise For Life Institute

A New Age of Fitness

Stephen G. Banks

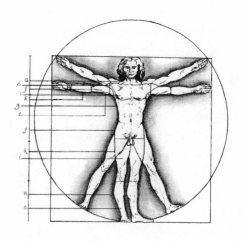

"   *The 1980's were the decade of* *"*
aerobic exercise. But still, many
of us can't lug the vacuum
upstairs without help. Which
brings us to the 1990's and a new
concept in exercise designed to
produce a new concept in fitness:
"balanced fitness."

Stephen G. Banks *is the editor and Publications Manager for The National Exercise For Life Institute. He is responsible for the publication of* Personal Fitness & Weight Loss *and* Active American *magazines in addition to a variety of books and newsletters. He has written and edited books and numerous feature articles on health related subjects including exercise, nutrition, weight control, stress, aging, and strength training. His work has been published in both the United States and Japan.*

1

Don't you hate asking people to open the peanut butter jar (move the TV, mow the grass, carry the suitcase, lift that box of stuff)? Don't you hate patting children on the head instead swinging them onto your shoulder, lugging groceries one bag at a time instead of two, driving a golf ball ten yards less every year instead of five yards more. Don't you just hate that? Of course. So does everybody else. At best it's embarrassing to be unable or uncomfortable doing everyday tasks. At worst it's annoying, dangerous and unhealthy.

The 1980's were the decade of aerobic exercise. En masse, we charged running paths, health clubs, the basement in a revolution against fat, cholesterol, and other maladies of poor cardiovascular conditioning. And it worked. Those of us who regularly do some type of aerobic exercise are thinner, trimmer, and healthier as a result. But still, many of us can't lug the vacuum upstairs without help. Which brings us to the 1990's and a new concept in exercise designed to produce a new concept in fitness: "balanced fitness."

The purpose of balanced fitness is to enhance the quality of a person's life by providing both health and the strength and stamina necessary to participate in a full and active lifestyle. In other words, balanced fitness is a slim, trim you with a healthy heart and a mean serve on the tennis court. It is achieved through a cross-training program of regular aerobic exercise and strength training.

Great, just great. A couple of thousand hours, a couple of thousand dollars worth of aerobic exercise equipment, and three dozen pairs of exercise shoes, and now you need to lift weights to be healthy. Forget it.

Get a porter to carry the suitcase.

Now just read this out. For the most part, cardiovascular (aerobic) exercises condition the systems responsible for transporting oxygen to the body: the heart, the lungs, the circulatory system. And it must be the basis of every exercise program since the benefits it provides -- weight control, energy, stamina -- are fundamentally essential to health and quality of life. Which means that all the sweat equity you've invested has been worth the effort.

The problem is, most forms of aerobic exercise don't build muscle strength, particularly in the upper body. Yet in terms of enhancing quality of day-to-day life, strength training may provide more noticeable benefits than aerobic exercise forms. As Neil McCartney of McMaster University in Ontario puts it, "After all, the average person doesn't often utilize 75% of his aerobic capacity, which running may demand. But he digs in the garden, carries luggage, totes grocery bags, picks up a tool box, saws wood. A human being characteristically works at very high levels for short intervals and rests, stopping and starting up again. It only makes sense that we should be training people to improve in the kind of work they actually do."

No way, right? You're not going to start throwing a sweaty barbell around your basement just to get at the peanut butter. It'd be a lot less work to buy the stuff in a plastic container with a snap-off top.

True. But only to a point. Substantial medical research now indicates that strength training, in addition to aerobic exercise, is an important component of maintaining overall health. This, they have discovered is true regardless of age, sex or fitness level. Like regular aerobic exercise, strength training helps condition the cardiovascular system. According to Dr. Linn Goldberg of Oregon Health Sciences University, "Weight training is not just a veneer. It can help cardiovascular health by reducing known risk factors, as well as help control body fat."

Competitive body builders, Dr. Goldberg found, experience the same improvements in cholesterol levels as long distance runners: a rise in HDL or "good" cholesterol, and a drop in LDL or "bad" cholesterol. In another study, Steven J. Fleck, Ph.D. and William J. Kraemer, Ph.D. found that competitive body builders had a more favorable cholesterol profile even than distance runners.

Strength training also helps control body weight, particularly in combination with aerobic exercise. Most of the calories consumed by the body are consumed by muscle. Losing muscle mass or allowing muscles to become weak and fatty reduces their ability to utilize calories. On the other hand, muscles that are exercised regularly burn calories quickly and efficiently.

That efficiency continues long after the exercise has been completed. In a comparison done between cycling (an aerobic exercise) and weight lifting, Goldberg found a 36% increase in caloric afterburn with strength training over the aerobic exercise.

Strength training can also help reduce the risk of osteoporosis and other diseases that cause bone loss. Current medical theory suggests that muscle activity stimulates the building of bone. In this application of strength training, the effectiveness of an exercise is contingent upon specificity. According to Dr. Barbara Drinkwater, former president of the American College of Sports Medicine (ACSM), "If you want an increase in density of the arm, stimulate the muscle pull on those bones."

Those are just a few of the health benefits of strength training. The lifestyle benefits are perhaps even more significant. Many medical professionals divide the human lifespan (very roughly) into three thirty year segments. For the first thirty years, balanced fitness is basically free. Muscle mass, aerobic endurance, and other physiological measures reach their peaks almost without effort.

It is during the second thirty years that balanced fitness through proper exercise and nutrition can make the most dramatic difference. In a sedentary person, aerobic endurance decreases at the rate of about one percent per year after approximately age thirty. Muscle mass decreases at about half that rate, three to six percent per decade. But, according to Dr. Donald Vickery of the Center for Corporate Health, a sixty-year-old person who exercises regularly can have the same bone density, muscle strength and mass, aerobic capacity, and other physiological attributes of a thirty-year-old. That's thirty years of life at peak fitness!

The third thirty year segment is a period of natural decline. Here, too, exercise plays a vital role in maintaining health and quality of life. Many if not most of the physiological changes attributed to aging are actually the result of sedentary living. According to Dr. Walter Bortz of the Palo Alto Medical Clinic in California, "Most of what passes as aging is not really aging, but disuse. 'Use it or lose it' is no longer just a conviction; it's absolutely riveted in science now."

Which is not to suggest that if you're sixty-years-old and have never exercised that there's no point in starting now. Quite the contrary. The people who achieve the greatest physiological and lifestyle benefits are those who have never exercised before. Study after study has shown that with regular exercise people in their eighties and even beyond can achieve significant improvements across a broad range of physiological measures including muscle strength, bone mass, and aerobic capacity!

The conviction that strength training should be a component of every exercise program is such that the ACSM is revising its widely followed fitness guidelines. Due to be released this April, the new guidelines are expected to recommend that in addition to a regular program of aerobic exercise, adults of all ages do some form of strength training exercise at least twice each week.

Convinced? Great. Back to "balanced fitness." The basic prescription for aerobic fitness was perhaps the most widely heralded medical advice of the 1980's: three or four times per week, perform any exercise (preferably a low- or no-impact activity) that raises the heart rate to 60 to 85 percent of its maximum and holds it there for 20 minutes.

The prescription for strength training while not yet as widely publicized, is no more complex: stress a muscle beyond its normal demands and it will react. If the intensity of the exercise is increased gradually, that reaction will be positive and the muscle will grow stronger. Instruments designed to provide that stress fall into basically two categories: free weights and resistance machines. Free weights, dumbbells and barbells, are probably the most recognized strength training devices. They are relatively inexpensive and lend themselves to a large number of exercises. Problems with them include the space required to use them, and safety. Proper supervision and instruction, particularly for beginners, are essential in any exercise program using free weights.

Resistance machines fall into several categories, each with its own advantages and disadvantages. Isotonic machines are designed to maintain a constant resistance throughout the range of motion and are relatively easy to use. The disadvantage is that they have some of the same safety problems as free weight exercises and that they are relatively expensive.

Variable resistance and "cam" machines are designed to alter resistance through the range of motion in order to maximize the load on the muscle and thus maximize the effect of the exercise. While this theory is appealing, most research studies have found that these devices are no more effective than conventional isotonic equipment.

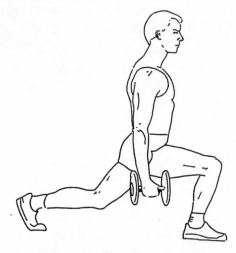

Proper supervision and instruction, particularly for beginners, are essential in any exercise program using free weights.

Isokinetic equipment limits the speed of the exercise and thereby provide resistance. These machines offer several important advantages. Like variable resistance and "cam" machines, they provide resistance according to muscle strength through the entire range of motion. They're safe since there is no actual weight involved. And they adjust automatically to each user's strength and fitness level.

The disadvantage of isokinetic machines has always been price since typically they could provide only one training modality per unit. Though today, with moderately priced equipment such as the Nordic Fitness Chair by NordicTrack available, this is no longer a consideration. This interesting machine's unique speed-sensitive resistance device and versatility make it immediately compatible with the fitness needs of every user. When it's not in use, it makes

Isokinetic equipment, like the Nordic Fitness Chair, provides resistance according to muscle strength through the entire range of motion.

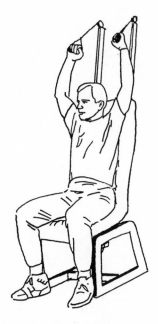

a handsome sidechair since its compact size, attractive oak and brushed nylon finish, and multiple colors match the decor of nearly any home.

In 1982, Dr. Kenneth Cooper published a book titled *The Aerobics Program for Total Well-Being* which went on to become the definitive work for the aerobics movement of the 1980's. The book begins, "One of the great principles of the universe is the principle of balance....And so it is with our bodies....And where there is perfect balance, there is what I call total well-being." Those words are as true today as they were then. Balance in all things, balanced fitness achieved through aerobic exercise and strength training, is an essential element of total well-being.

The Equal Strength Amendment: Strength Training For Women

Gordon Bakoulis Bloch

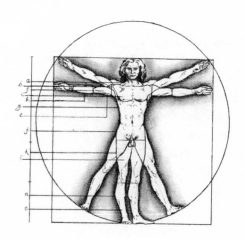

66 *Most women who design a* 99
*moderate strength training
program find that over time, they
develop a trimmer, sleeker look.*

Gordon Bakoulis Bloch *is a freelance writer in New York
City and former editor of* Health *magazine. She has
written and edited numerous feature articles and columns
for major periodicals on the subjects of health, personal
fitness, nutrition and weight control. She is a competitive
long-distance runner with national class times, has com-
peted in the U.S. Olympic marathon trials, and has been
selected as the Big Apple Runner of the Year.*

2

Congratulations. You're a woman who has integrated fitness into a healthy, productive life. You manage to squeeze in some sort of aerobic exercise -- jogging, swimming, a class, a machine workout -- for at least 20 to 30 minutes, three times a week. As a result you feel more vigorous, you maintain your weight, and are better able to cope with life's daily stresses. Want to play touch football with your kids, take a weekend hike with friends, dash a block to catch the bus? No problem.

Now, if only you could get the lid off the peanut butter jar.

A generation ago, a woman wasn't expected to be strong enough to unscrew a stubborn lid, uncork a wine bottle, unstick a tight water faucet, or carry a suitcase. After all, women didn't exercise and were considered frail and helpless -- the "weaker sex." Besides, it was considered perfectly appropriate, even expected, to turn such tasks over to the nearest male (who probably was not more aerobically fit -- he simply had a bit more bicep).

Times have changed. Women are expected and encouraged to take matters (and jars) into their own hands, and any man who happens to be around to help will likely be sensitive enough to female equality not to lend his muscle until the lady in question has practically put her arm in a sling.

In other words, a woman these days would do well to get strong -- to train her muscles to lift, lower, push and pull more weight than she can at her present level. Traditionally, this has involved working with weights (either free or machines) or the weight of the body. Such routines have also traditionally been the province of men, who grunted and strained and lifted heavy loads in grimy gyms and weight rooms, "pumping iron" to emulate Arnold Schwarzenegger. But the recent shift in the fitness movement to a more moderate effort has cast strength training in a new light. "People realize they don't have to spend hours a week in the weight room to get strong," says Greg Niederlander, MS, educational coordinator of personalized training at the Multiplex Fitness Club in Deerfield, Illinois. That can be particularly attractive to women, many of whom don't want big, bulky muscles anyway. "Most women are looking for a toned, sculpted look -- to them, big muscles have a negative stigma."

There's evidence that large numbers of women are trying strength training these days. Although women accounted for only 17.5% of the $184 million Americans spent on home weight-lifting equipment in 1988, they spent almost half the total dollars shelled out for workout/fitness shoes (the kind most people use to strength-train), according to the National Sporting Goods Association. Neil Wolkodoff, MS, sports sciences director of the Denver Athletic Club, says that the number of women strength training at the club has doubled over the past three years. Niederlander, who works as a personal trainer, says most of his new strength-training clients are female.

Muscle Benefits

There are a number of reasons why strength training can be valuable to women -- many of which also apply to men. Probably the most important is that strength training helps provide balanced fitness. An aerobic program strengthens your heart, which can reduce your risk of heart disease and raise your energy level. Most aerobic activities also build muscle endurance, the ability to repeat less-than-full-strength contractions or to sustain a single moderate contraction. As a result, any activity that uses the endurance-trained muscles (including the heart) can be performed for a longer period. But to build strength, the maximal force a muscle can exert at one time, you must strength train, or accustom muscles to working intensely for brief periods. This "overload" -- working the muscle to the point where it can't sustain a contraction any longer -- adds to the proportion of muscle that generates a contraction, and this makes muscle stronger.

Strong muscles make you better equipped to handle a myriad of daily tasks -- from lugging home a full briefcase to swinging a child overhead in play. "You'll enjoy life more by enabling your body to carry on daily activities in a comfortable zone," says Niederlander.

Strength is also protection against injury, both in fitness activities and daily life, according to Wayne Westcott, Ph.D., strength consultant for the National YMCA and fitness director of the South Shore YMCA in Quincy, Massachusetts. Although studies were scarce (injuries occur for many different reasons, and it's hard to control for them all), it's known that strength training not only makes muscles stronger, but also strengthens tendons, ligaments and bones. Strong muscles also protect joints -- a strong quadricep (front of thigh) muscle cushions the knee, for example. "If you think of the body as a car, strong muscles are the shock absorbers," says Westcott. Muscles that are strong enough to take the pounding of high-impact activities are especially helpful in preventing injuries among runners, dancers and players in sports such as soccer, basketball and field hockey. But anyone who is active -- whose muscles are called into play beyond the scope of sedentary living -- will likely reduce her injury risk regardless of the activity. You're also less likely to get hurt in daily activities -- turning, bending, reaching -- especially if you strengthen the back, shoulder, and abdominal muscles, which are called into play in almost every action imaginable.

Psychological Strength, Too

Strength training gains extend beyond the physiological into the realm of the psychological. One study of college-age men found that those who were more muscularly fit were more confident, emotionally stable and outgoing. The results are perhaps even more applicable to women. "With strength training, you see progress in a very real, tangible form," notes Wolkodoff. Women, who are less likely than men to have developed strength in other activities, may see more impressive initial gains. It wouldn't be unusual, he says, for a woman to increase the strength of large muscles in her legs, arms, shoulder and back by 20-40% over a period of six to eight weeks. This increase in strength pays off in a broad range of psychological benefits important to women, including greater self-confidence and esteem.

Getting Stronger Without Bulk

As mentioned before, most women would rather not acquire bulk along with their strength. Fortunately, there's little reason to worry. That's because women have very little of the male hormone testosterone which is what enables men -- along with intense training -- to acquire massive bodybuilder's physiques. "I have women clients who could work out like football players and they'd never build bulk," says Niederlander, who has worked as a strength consultant for the Texas Rangers, Cincinnati Reds, Chicago White Sox and Chicago Bulls. Building bulk is also a matter of genetics: Women <u>and</u> men who have gangly builds won't get bulky muscles no matter how hard they train.

It's unlikely that the average woman will be able to lift as much as the average man, since strength is proportional to muscle size. Women tend to have a greater percentage of body fat than men -- and therefore a smaller percentage of muscle -- which limits their potential strength gains. However, Westcott points out that male and female muscle fiber look identical under the microscope and respond in exactly the same way to the strength training stimulus. "In terms of muscle tissue, women are pound for pound as strong as men," he says. In fact, some studies have shown that women can achieve greater strength gains, proportionally, in certain muscles.

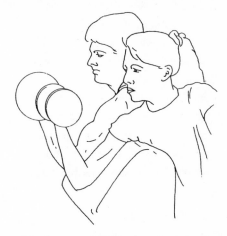

Because of the hormonal differences between women and men, most women need not worry about developing big, bulging muscles.

If you're still worried about bulk, Wolkodoff suggests taking note of how your legs respond to fairly strenuous weight-bearing activities such as jogging, basketball or racquet sports. If you develop a more muscular look than you care for, you might want to design a program that uses light weights for many repetitions. This builds more endurance than strength -- although the muscles will get stronger and slightly bulkier as well.

Most women who design a moderate strength training program find that over time, they develop a trimmer, sleeker look. That's because muscle is denser than fat. When you strength train, you're not "transforming" muscle into fat, but the result is likely more of the former and less of the latter. "Muscle is your best friend for weight control," says Westcott. That's because muscle burns calories at a faster rate than fat, and calories that aren't burned are stored on the body as fat. A strength training plan by itself (provided you don't overeat) will likely make you more toned, although your body weight may actually increase due to muscle's greater density. If you're interested in reducing body fat, it's best to combine a strength training routine with a program of moderate aerobic exercise, and follow a reasonable, low-fat, low-cholesterol diet. Getting regular aerobic exercise is a good idea anyway for maintaining cardiovascular health. Keep in mind that strength training cannot help you "spot-reduce" -- reduce fat in unwanted areas, such as thighs or stomach. The loss of subcutaneous fat -- the fat just below the surface of the skin -- takes place bodywide through a program of fat burning exercise and sensible eating.

Picking a Program

Deciding what kind of strength training program to embark on means taking a look at your fitness needs and goals, and assessing how much time and effort you're willing to put into a regular routine. A program does not have to be intensive or lengthy to be effective. Westcott recently completed a study of healthy but sedentary men and women in the Boston area who were put on a program of 20 minutes of exercise, three times a week. They worked out aerobically for 15 minutes, then strength trained for five minutes, working their leg, back, biceps and chest muscles. After eight weeks, they saw 20-25% strength gains in muscles exercised, along with gains of one to two pounds of muscle and losses of three to four pounds of fat. "This shows that even the briefest sessions are useful," says Westcott.

You may opt for longer and/or more frequent sessions, which is fine. Just make sure not to work the same muscles on two consecutive days, as muscle fiber needs about 48 hours to recover and consolidate gains made. Another workout before then, unless you are very highly trained, will just wear the muscles out and possibly cause injury. Also keep in mind that in general, lifting a light weight for many repetitions builds endurance, while heavy weights for fewer repetitions brings greater strength gains, which usually means greater muscle size, too. Muscle soreness when starting a strength training program is normal. If you feel joint pain, however, reduce your intensity and make sure you're using correct form.

Strength training does not reduce flexibility if muscles are worked through their full range of motion. The NordicPower provides constant resistance through the full range of motion.

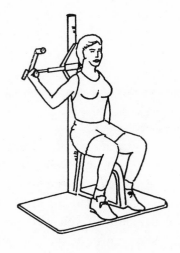

You may choose to strength train in a health club, or in the convenience of your home, with free weights or machines. And working out at home doesn't need to involve a lot of complicated equipment. The new NordicPower, by NordicTrack, not only works every major muscle group in your body, but is compact enough to store. It provides constant resistance through the full range of motion, so your muscles provide the power.

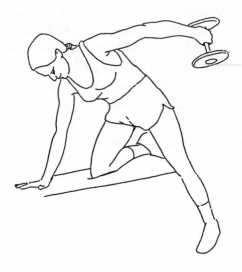

Women should take advantage of the wide range of choices available for strength training. Whatever method is chosen, proper technique and form should be followed to avoid injury and gain maximum benefits.

Whatever method you pick, learn proper technique to avoid injury and to make sure you work muscles through their full range of motion. Contrary to popular belief, strength training does not reduce flexibility if you work muscles through their range of motion, and warm up before and cool down after the workout. "I try to help my clients <u>increase</u> flexibility by building stronger muscles and connective tissue," says Neiderlander. Using isokinetic machines, which apply varied resistance at different parts of the lift, is one of the best ways to do this; if you don't have access to this type of equipment, your best strategy is to avoid lifting too-heavy weights.

Wolkodoff notes that some women are intimidated by the wide range of choices in weights, and adopt a limiting program as a result. "Women shouldn't be scared of free weights," he says. Consider a program that mixes training modes -- for example, using dumbbells, which are easy to grasp in your hands, for arms and shoulders, and machines for back, abdominals and lower body.

As more women consider strength training a part of balanced fitness, the experts predict that women's knowledge will increase and their concerns will become more sophisticated. Neiderlander sees this shift occurring already. "Most women I see <u>know</u> the many benefits of strength training," he says. "They know that high repetitions at a low weight builds tone. They know they can't spot-reduce. They're ready to make strength training a part of their lives."

Aerobic Exercise, Strength Training, and Bone Mass

Kenneth H. Cooper, M.D., M.P.H.
with Sydney Lou Bonnick, M.D.

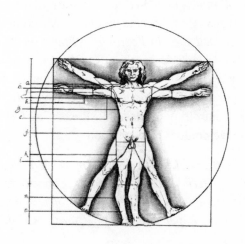

" Medical research has now proven "
that strength training can have
an extremely beneficial effect on
bone mass . . . and may play a
role in the prevention of
osteoporosis.

Kenneth H. Cooper, M.D., M.P.H., *is a recognized leader in health and fitness and Director of the Aerobics Center in Dallas, Texas. Dr. Cooper is the author of* Aerobics, *the book that started the cardiovascular fitness movement. His other books include* Aerobics for Women, The Aerobics Way, The New Aerobics, Running Without Fear, *and three volumes of Dr. Cooper's Preventive Medicine Program:* Controlling Cholesterol, Preventing Osteoporosis, *and* Overcoming Hypertension.

Sydney Lou Bonnick *is a graduate of the University of Texas Southwestern Medical School and is board-certified in Internal Medicine. She is Director of Osteoporosis Services at the Cooper Clinic at the Aerobics Center in Dallas, Texas.*

3

The importance of regular aerobic exercise is well known and documented. Weight reduction, improved cardiovascular performance, improved lung function, and an overall increase in both physical and emotional well-being are just a few of the many benefits of a regular aerobic workout. In fact, in 1978, the American College of Sports Medicine basically equated fitness with aerobic exercise by recommending aerobic exercise 3 to 5 days per week for 15 to 60 minutes for all healthy adults. However, that recommendation made no reference to strength training.

In the last few years the benefits of strength training have been closely examined. While many considered strength training only in terms of increased muscle bulk, the benefits of strength training are now known to be far more extensive. Medical research has now proven that strength training can have an extremely beneficial effect on bone mass as well as muscle. In the past, women have often avoided strength training because of a perceived social bias against developed muscle mass in women. But the benefits for women far outweigh the social stigma because of the role that strength training may play in the prevention of osteoporosis. This is one of the reasons that the American College of Sports Medicine has just amended its 1978 recommendations to include two strength training sessions per week in addition to 3 to 5 aerobic workouts.

Osteoporosis is a disorder of the bone which currently affects some 24 million Americans. The disease causes gradual bone loss which can eventually result in bone fractures with little or no trauma. Statistically, 1 out of every 3 women in their 60's will suffer a fracture in the spine because of osteoporosis, and one out of every 3 women in their 70's will break her hip.

The treatment of osteoporosis remains very difficult at best. There is no question that the best approach is to prevent it, and one of the most effective means of prevention is to develop the maximum bone mass possible prior to the onset of bone loss and then to maintain the bone to the highest degree possible. This is where the benefits of strength training on bone mass are just beginning to be realized.

The strength of the skeleton is predominantly determined by the amount of mineral in the bone, which is referred to as bone mineral density. For all practical purposes, the terms bone mass, bone density and bone strength can be used synonymously.

Although bone is often thought of as a hard, inert substance, it actually has a life cycle of its own. During this life cycle, old bone is destroyed, then replaced. In order to increase in height during the growth years, more bone must obviously be made than is destroyed. But even after an individual reaches maximum height, density can continue to increase. Left to its own devices, bone will reach its maximum density level sometime during a person's twenties and almost certainly prior to the age of 30. There is generally no additional increase in density unless specific measures are taken to stimulate the metabolism of the bone. After age 40, a decline in bone density is often seen in both men and women, ultimately resulting in sufficient loss of density to compromise bone strength. It is at this point that fractures of the spine, hip and wrists often occur. Frequently, these occur, not because of some serious accident, but simply during the course of every day activities.

While inherited factors certainly play a role in the development of maximum height and bone density, lifestyle factors such as exercise clearly influence the development of bone strength. The potential benefits of exercise on bone mass include the initial development of a higher peak bone density prior to age 30, the maintenance of any given level of bone density after the usual age of attainment of peak bone mass, and the ability to increase bone density after the usual age of attainment of peak bone mass.

Along with the many other exciting revelations from the NASA space program, the effect of weightlessness on bone mass reinforced the belief that exercise is important in the maintenance of bone strength. Using techniques which allowed scientists to measure the bone density of the astronauts of Skylab 4 both before and after space flight, it was discovered that weightlessness caused a marked loss of bone strength. In the absence of the pull of gravity, the bones were no longer required to support the weight of the body. As a consequence, the bones began to deteriorate rapidly. The calcium that was lost from the bones was eliminated from the body through the kidneys in such large amounts that there was actually concern that the astronauts might develop kidney stones in space! NASA's original plans for providing exercise for astronauts in space had centered around providing aerobic exercise to maintain cardiovascular fitness, which can easily be done in zero gravity. They are now working to devise forms of strength training that can be performed in space in order to protect the astronauts from muscle and bone deterioration.

Research on the effects of various types of exercise on the bones for those of us who are earth-bound is also proceeding. Much of this research has been done in just the last ten years because only recently has the sophisticated technology been developed to measure bone density. As early as 1971 however, research was published in Sweden in which the bone density of the lower leg was measured in three different groups of men: professional or world

class amateur athletes, recreational athletes and those who participated in no regular exercise at all. The types of exercise performed
by these various groups included weight lifting, running, soccer
and swimming.

The findings from this early study indicate that the professional athletes and world class amateurs had significantly stronger
lower leg bones than the recreational athletes and non-exercising
men. But the recreational athlete had stronger leg bone than the
non-exercisers. When the effects of the different types of exercise
on the leg bone were examined, the activities which produced the
greatest load on the leg resulted in the stronger leg and the greater
bone density. The weight lifters had the strongest leg bones,
followed by the runners and soccer players, and then the swimmers.
This suggested that even the modest exercise programs performed
by the recreational athletes could increase bone strength, but the
exercises which created the greatest load on the bone were potentially the most effective in increasing bone strength.

In support of this theory were two other early studies looking
at specific types of exercise. In 1980 results were published on a
group of male tennis players. The bone strength in both forearms
was measured in these men. The strength of the bone in the racket
arm, which had been subjected to the repetitive impact of the tennis
ball hitting the racket, was much greater than that found in the non-
racket arm. In the latter part of 1980's , the technology for measur-
ing bone strength in the spine became available and researchers
began to look at the effects of loading on this area of the skeleton.
A study of power lifters in Sweden utilized this new technology to
examine the effects of lifting on the spine. The study showed that
the power lifters had greater bone strength in the lower spine than
a similar group of men who were not power lifters.

Of course, most of us are not power lifters, nor are we world
class athletes, although we may aspire to be. There are many studies

now examining the effects of recreational running and fitness regimens using resistance machines and free weights on bone strength. In a study performed by researchers at the Stanford University School of Medicine in 1986, male and female runners were found to have 40% more bone mass than their non-running counterparts. In 1989, at the University of South Carolina, muscle building exercises performed with free weights and resistance machines were shown to increase bone strength in men. In a combined study at several medical institutions in Texas in 1990, women who regularly engaged in strength training using resistance machines were able to increase their bone strength, while the bone strength of their non-exercising peers declined. Collectively, these studies indicate that weight bearing activities like running and strength training exercises using free weights and resistance machines can increase bone mass in both men and women in the spine, arms and legs. Strength training exercises have a greater effect on the bone than purely weight bearing exercise. However, the strongest bones were found in those men and women who participated in a balanced fitness program involving both aerobic and strength training exercises. The benefits were not only seen in young men and women, increases in bone strength were seen after such exercise programs in participants who were in their seventies!

Other studies have looked at the ability to predict bone strength from levels of physical activity in general and aerobic fitness and muscle strength specifically. Researchers have found that increasing levels of physical activity in general is highly predictive of increased bone strength. Increased bone strength can also be predicted independently from both aerobic fitness, as measured by maximal oxygen uptake during a stress test and muscle strength, as measured on an isokinetic dynamometer in participants ranging in age from 20 to 75.

Clearly, both aerobic and strength training exercise can increase bone strength. In the last twenty years men and women of all ages who participated in a variety of exercise regimens have been studied to determine the effects of those regimens on bone strength. As the technology which allows us to study the bones has become more sophisticated, our knowledge of the effects of exercise on the skeleton has also become more sophisticated.

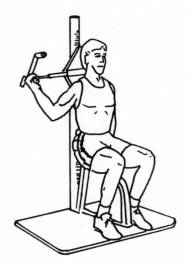

Resistance machines like the NordicPower can increase bone mass in both men and women. However, a balanced fitness program including both strength training and aerobic exercise will provide the greatest degree of bone strength.

While aerobic exercise has long been viewed as a means to cardiovascular fitness, it is also a means to increased bone mass <u>and</u> strength. Strength training, considered by some as only a means to larger muscle mass and enhanced appearance, may well be the most valuable form of exercise for increasing bone mass in both men and women. And as such, it becomes an extremely valuable tool in the prevention of osteoporosis and the preservation of health and quality of life.

The Anti-Aging Art of
Strength Training

Robert K. Cooper, Ph.D.

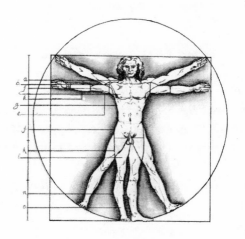

"   *No matter whether you're 40 or*   *"*
80 right now, you can prevent or
reverse many effects of aging --
and exercise is one of the best
places to begin.

Robert K. Cooper, Ph.D., *author of* Health & Fitness Excellence: The Comprehensive Action Plan, *is a nationally certified instructor for leading preventive medicine organizations. He is certified as a Health and Fitness Instructor by the American College of Sports Medicine, and serves on the advisory board of the* Living Well *media series. Dr. Cooper is the director of the Center for Health and Fitness Excellence, an educational institute in Minnesota.*

4

Once you reach adulthood, your muscles and mind begin a slow predictable, downhill course. Or at least that's what conventional wisdom says. Yet worldwide research shows this is far from inevitable. No matter whether you're 40 or 80 right now, you can prevent or reverse many effects of aging -- and exercise is one of the best places to begin.

Beyond Aerobics
It Takes Strength to Live a Long, Vigorous Life

When most Americans think of exercise, they think of *aerobics*, including walking, jogging, cycling, cross-country skiing, dance-exercise, swimming, and rowing. While aerobic exercise generally tops the list in terms of importance to your heart and lungs, it makes only a limited contribution to building muscle, especially in the torso or upper body, and it's not enough to create what experts call *balanced fitness* -- which is developed through a combination of aerobics and strength training.

More than four hundred muscles make your body firm -- or let it sag. If these muscles aren't made strong and balanced in relationship to each other -- and kept that way -- they slowly wither away as time goes by. For years, scientists have known that muscular strength improves posture, helps prevent back pain, and is the foundation of lifelong physical skill, coordination, and balance.

New research shows that simple strength-building exercises also improve cardiovascular health, help prevent osteoporosis, reduce excess body fat, and may even sharpen the mind.

"The need for maintaining muscular strength and endurance is important at all age levels," says John Piscopo, Ph.D., professor at the State University of New York at Buffalo, and author of *Fitness and Aging.* "However, this fitness component has special meaning for older persons because it is the source of energy and force necessary for the maintenance of good posture and proficient movement skills, as well as a protective buffer for bones and soft tissues."

"Strength training is not just a veneer," says Dr. Linn Goldberg of Oregon Health Sciences University in Portland, whose studies have shown that, for both men and women, strength training can improve blood cholesterol levels, burn fat, and provide good "adaptation" -- a cardiovascular response that reduces blood pressure and heart rate. It's even possible for 60- or 70-year-olds who exercise regularly to have the same muscle tone, posture, flexibility, resting heart rate, and blood pressure they had at age 25 or 35.

In a major new study published in the *Journal of the American Medical Association*, researchers report that even a minimal amount of regular exercise confers significant protection not only from cardiovascular disease but also against death from a wide range of other causes. This increases the evidence that exercise may help ward off cancer -- a relationship discovered only in the past few years.

You may also be surprised to learn that osteoporosis -- the thinning-bones condition commonly associated with women -- can also be a serious problem for men. Recent studies published in the *Annals of Internal Medicine* and the journal *Age* show that men, too, experience significant bone loss as they age. Strength training is an excellent form of exercise to help prevent -- or reverse -- this damage.

In addition, research shows that regular exercise sharpens mental abilities -- reasoning, memory, and reaction time -- of people from their late 40's on. "Someone over age 50 who exercises regularly has more energy, has a better sex life, and can work longer hours than someone who doesn't," says Dr. James Fries, an epidemiologist at Stanford University.

Advantages of being physically active

This graph shows that a physically active person has about a 20 year advantage over a sedentary person in terms of function. Note that the treadmill time of a 65 year old active person is about the same as the sedentary 45 year old.*

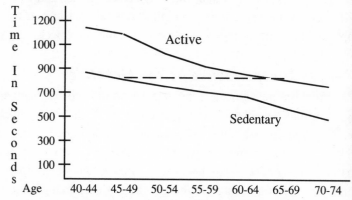

* Results from the analysis of maximal treadmill test performance in more than 4,000 men examined at the Cooper Clinic, Dallas, Texas.

Equally Important for Men and Women

Muscle strengthening exercises are just as vital for women as they are for men, says Dr. Barbara Drinkwater, president of the

American College of Sports Medicine. "It's healthy that women are now accepting muscles as part of a normal human body."

For both sexes, the basic fact of strength training is simple: Stress your muscles by making them work against resistance and they'll get stronger to meet the challenge. Muscles respond immediately -- and at any age -- so each of us has the lifelong capacity to develop more strength and tone.

When it comes to muscles, the only difference between male and female is size. The sex hormone testosterone plays a key role in muscle growth, and men have more of this biochemical than women. On similar strength training programs, male muscle fibers will increase in mass long after a female's have stopped growing (there's absolutely no truth to the idea that, for women, getting stronger means getting "huge" muscles). But *both* men and women will continue to build more strength -- due at least in part to an improved nervous system activation of the muscle fibers.

A Key to Independence as You Get Older

From middle age on, strong muscles provide you with advantages you may never have given them credit for. With healthy, well-toned muscles, your body is balanced, better coordinated, and more vibrant. You can do more of what you want wherever you want to do it. By easing the tasks of daily life -- toting grocery bags, raising windows, carrying luggage, digging in the garden, picking up tools, wrestling with the grandchildren, bounding up stairs -- muscular strength and endurance constantly contribute to your independence and well-being.

When you strengthen your muscles you improve both *absolute* strength (the ability to lift a weight once) and *muscular endurance* (the ability to repeat a muscular contraction many times in quick succession). Strong muscles reinforce the joints they support, so that you're much less likely to experience common aches and pains -- or to strain your shoulders, elbows, knees, or back. And endurance allows muscles to make a sustained effort, which in day-to-day life means greater resistance to fatigue.

Eight Basic Guidelines for Strength Training

Once you've been cleared by your doctor to begin a moderate strength-building fitness program, it pays to learn how "exercising smarter" can give you better results and do it faster. For example, many people assume that developing strong, toned muscles requires dozens of exercises. The truth is, it doesn't. If you select some good basic exercises and do them correctly, you will quickly feel and see the improvement. Here are some basic guidelines:

1. Decide How Much Time You're Willing to Spend.

Option 1: The Bare Minimum. If you feel especially pressed for time, your first question is probably not, How much do I need to do? but rather, How little can I get away with?

The key here is to take a look at what strength benefits you may already be receiving from other parts of your fitness program and then choose the fastest, easiest ways to take care of those muscles not yet being toned.

(a) Choose aerobic exercises that help build strength and endurance in the greatest number of body areas. Some of the most effective upper-body/lower-body aerobic activities are (alphabetically): cross-country skiing; integrated stationary cycling (with arm resistance from moving levers); rowing; swimming; and walking/jogging with light hand/wrist weights.

(b) Find ways to strengthen the major muscle areas you don't reach with (a) above. Select weekend/holiday recreational activities where you use your muscles to step, turn, reach, lift, rotate, push, and pull in different ways from your regular aerobic exercise.

Option 2: More Comprehensive Strength and Endurance

Training. For best overall fitness, at some point you'll want to take strength training at least one step further. If you choose a routine wisely, the maximum time you probably need to spend is about 25-30 minutes four days a week. The exercises may be performed without equipment (using body-weight resistance, for example) or with equipment (rubber tubing, dumbbells, barbells, or machine weights).

If you are over age 40 and starting a strength training program, I strongly advise against doing certain popular exercises: squats, straight-leg sit-ups or leg lifts, toe touches, deep knee bends, bench presses with a bar, deadlifts, behind-the-neck presses with a bar, and bent-over rowing with a bar.

A complete, illustrated strength-training program is included in my book *Health & Fitness Excellence: The Comprehensive Action Plan* (Houghton Mifflin, 1990). If you don't currently belong to a fitness center or own a multipurpose home strength-training machine, or if before investing in either of these options you want to try a simple, streamlined home program, I recommend the following basic exercises (which can be performed with a set of dumbbells, two sturdy chairs, a flat bench, and ankle weights): *Chest* -- modified push-ups, modified dips, and dumbbell flyes; *Shoulders* -- side lateral dumbbell raises and upright dumbbell rowing; *Arms* -- bicep dumbbell curls, arm extensions, and triceps press-downs; *Back* -- modified bent-over dumbbell rowing and modified dips; *Abdomen* -- "transpyramid" breathing, abdominal roll-ups, and reverse trunk rotations; *Thighs* -- modified half-knee bends, outer thigh lifts, inner thigh lifts, and leg extensions; *Calves* -- toe raises and toe taps.

2. Choose a Sensible Personal Training Schedule.

The most important rule in strength exercises is start easy. A *repetition* ("rep") is an individual full cycle of an exercise; for example, a traditional bicep curling exercise requires that the weight in your hands (palms out, arms down at a level below the waist) is raised (bending the arms at the elbow) from about mid-thigh level up to the front of the shoulder and back down to the starting position. The whole motion is a single repetition. A *set* is a group of repetitions performed in sequence. As a general guideline for beginners, one of two sets are recommended, each with between 6 and 12 repetitions of every exercise.

Let's say you initially choose two exercises for each major body area. Select your starting point (the chest, for example) and, once you've warmed up, go through 6-12 repetitions of chest exercise number 1. Select the proper resistance so that you can do at least 6 reps but not more than 12 before your muscles are temporarily so fatigued that you can't make another proper contraction. Your muscles will feel like they've worked hard, but safely. Then move on to the second chest exercise and go through 6-12 reps. This completes the first set. Rest for 60 to 90 seconds -- or long enough to let your breathing return to normal while you focus your mind on the next set of exercises (for the shoulders, for example). Then proceed with the workout.

Note: After being intensively exercised, muscles need at least 48 hours -- and sometimes 72 hours -- of rest and recovery. Therefore, some authorities suggest performing all of the upper-body exercises (chest, shoulders, back, and arms) in one workout -- for example, on Monday and Thursday; and all of the abdominal and leg exercises in a separate workout -- on Tuesday and Friday.

3. Precede Each Workout with a Warm-up -- and Don't Stretch.

Contrary to popular belief, stretching before a workout does not reduce injuries and may even be harmful -- causing tiny tears in tendons and ligaments and weakening joint structure. Proper strength-building exercises make your body more flexible, rather

than less.The ideal warm-up starts with comfortable movement --
usually a slower, less vigorous version of your upcoming fitness
activity -- that increases your heart rate and warms the inside temperature of your muscles several degrees -- which does help prevent
injuries.

4. Pay Attention to Safety.

Beyond a good warm-up, other strength training safety tips
include wearing good-fitting athletic shoes with nonskid soles and
comfortable clothes that hug the body enough not to get snagged on
equipment; working out with an exercise partner to boost motivation; and following each workout with a cool-down period.

5. Use Proper Form and Full Range-of-Motion.

A good exercise allows you to move the muscle through its
full range of motion, since partial movement can cause uneven

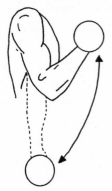

*Be sure to move the
muscle through its
full range of motion.*

strengthening or restrict the flexibility of your joints.

Since proper form and intensity are so important in strength-
building exercises, it's a good idea to consider working with a
qualified instructor, especially during the first few weeks of a new
program. But if you opt for one-on-one guidance, choose it wisely.

Never assume that a "staff member" shirt or a good physique signify professional competence.

The most qualified fitness instructors are usually certified (through comprehensive practical and written examinations) by one or more of the following organizations: American College of Sports Medicine (P.O. Box 1440, Indianapolis, IN 46206); Institute for Aerobics Research (12330 Preston Rd., Dallas, TX 75230); or the National Strength and Conditioning Association (P.O. Box 81410, Lincoln, NE 68501).

6. Exercise Slowly and Steadily.

Avoid fast or sudden movements -- which can cause injury. Exercise with smooth, controlled motions, keep breathing steadily, and never hold your breath longer than a second or two since this can restrict blood returning to the heart.

7. Use the Overload Principle.

The only way to tone or strengthen a muscle is to place a greater-then-normal demand on it -- that is, to overload it. As your muscles grow stronger, you must progressively increase the exercise resistance to keep improving.

8. Cool Down Gradually.

Abruptly stopping a workout can cause blood to pool in the veins, creating a sudden change in blood pressure and stress on the heart. After you've completed your workout, keep moving for at least three or four minutes to let your body gradually return to a non-exercising state.

Conclusion

Exercise is a cornerstone of a long, healthy, productive life. "Despite the millions that we spend on creams, supplements, formulas, and diets that are purported to turn back the clock," writes New York Times personal health columnist Jane E. Brody, "exercise is the only 'potion' that comes close to being a true fountain of youth."

Even in moderate amounts, strength training exercises will give you a new surge of vitality -- and help improve the way you look, feel, think, and perform. As your strength increases, you'll unlock an inner sense of confidence and body wisdom that cannot be drawn forth in any other way. And this, in turn, will put you in closer touch -- at every age -- with life's wonders and rewards.

Why Weight?
Strength Training in the 1990's

Marty Duda

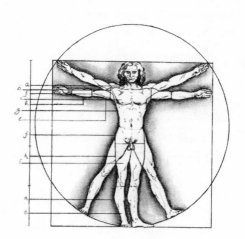

"   *Strength training should be*   **"**
viewed as the perfect complement
to aerobic training in creating
balanced fitness, the essence of
health, beauty and quality of life.

Marty Duda *is a freelance writer from St. Paul, MN who has written extensively on the health and safety aspects of sports and exercise, including* Family Safety and Health *magazine of the National Safety Council in Chicago. He is also a former writer and editor for* The Physician and Sportsmedicine *journal.*

5

For two decades, aerobic exercise has been the byword of fitness. And rightly so. Research has proven again and again the benefits of continuous, rhythmic exercise such as swimming, walking, running, cross-country skiing, and biking, and it has firmly established aerobic conditioning as the foundation for health and cardiovascular fitness.

But somehow lost in the hype for 30-minute jogs and 20-minute jaunts to nowhere on indoor exercise machines has been the importance of strength training. Perhaps strength training has suffered a negative image from competitive bodybuilders, fanatical weight lifters, and others who demonstrate the extremes. As a result, the vast majority of fitness buffs either are intimidated by bulging biceps, or want to disassociate themselves from programs that flaunt all that muscle. However, strength training need not be excessive and can be the key to creating that trim, tapered look that has become so popular. Indeed, strength training should be viewed as the perfect complement to aerobic training in creating balanced fitness, the essence of health, beauty and quality of life.

"The human body is an amazing machine and it needs a total fitness program," says Dean Brittenham, director of the Center for Athletic Development at the National Institute for Fitness and Sports in Indianapolis. "Strength training is one integral part of the fitness pie that helps determine how long this machine lasts. The body is designed to last 140 years, but we proceed to destroy it by lack of development, lack of use, or lack of maintenance. The thing that wears out fastest is the heart, so that should be the focus of exercise programs. Of course the heart is affected by other factors such as diet. But to exercise the heart muscle best we need to develop the entire muscular system surrounding it."

What is Strength Training?

Developing the muscular system means different things for different people. For the competitive weight lifter, it means grunting and groaning with eyes bulging to thrust 500 pounds overhead in a single lift. But for the average active American, sufficient strength gains can be achieved with less ambitious and more health-conscious goals.

According to the National Strength and Conditioning Association (NSCA), "Strength training is the use of progressive resistance methods to increase one's ability to exert or resist force. This type of training may utilize free weights, the individual's own body weight, machines, or other devices to attain this goal. In order to be measurably effective, the training sessions must include timely progressions in intensity, which provides sufficient demands to stimulate strength gains that are greater than those associated with normal growth and development."

So, according to that definition, strength training, which essentially is synonymous with the term "resistance training," can be any method used to resist or bear force, from push-ups to bench pressing your 2-year-old daughter to performing a quick, half-a-dozen exercises on NordicTrack's new Nordic Fitness Chair. This unique device uses the isokinetic principle to provide a complete, upper-body workout in as little as 10 minutes, right in the living area of your home.

"Weight training" is one type of strength training which in-

corporates the use of barbells, dumbbells, and machine-type appa-
ratuses as resistance. The terms "weight lifting" and "power
lifting" represent competitive sports that contest maximal lifting
ability, or how much weight one can lift in one attempt, or one
repetition.

Strength Training Benefits

Whatever the mode of exercise, strength training, if conducted correctly, will yield a broad range of benefits. Increased
muscle mass, strength and endurance, and enhanced flexibility are
the well-established physical benefits of strength training. But
because the systems of the body are so interrelated, it's hard to
measure the true value of strength training. Certainly a body with
strong, flexible muscles provides good framework for the all-
important aerobic exercise. However, documenting the benefits of
strength training specifically in terms of increased life span is difficult.

"You may not live an additional day by strength training, but
you will live a longer day -- or you'll experience a higher quality of
life for the years you do live," says Douglas M. Semenick, director
of the Faculty and Staff Wellness Program and a strength and conditioning coach at the University of Louisville.

Semenick offers numerous anecdotal accounts of the benefits
of strength training. "My father is 73 and he's been weight training
for 50 years; he's also a walker," says Semenick. "You'd probably
say he's in his late 50's if you saw him. He's developed and
maintained his strength and aerobic fitness. As a result, his quality
of life is so much higher than the typical man his age."

The body's natural aging process will probably be slowed
down if strength is developed and maintained, as demonstrated by
Semenick's father. By the time most people reach their 20's, their
resting metabolic rate (RMR -- the rate at which we burn calories

at rest) decreases. They become less active and start to lose muscle mass. As their RMR goes down and they consume a stable amount of calories, they are more apt to gain weight. The decreasing lean muscle mass and the corresponding increase in body fat contribute to the body's decline, making it difficult to burn carbohydrates and even more difficult to burn fat, which is the last energy source to be tapped.

As Brittenham puts it, "The human body is the only machine that gets better with use. The lower we keep our body fat, the more productive the human machine will be."

Everyday Living Enhanced

Indeed, strength gains will improve one's quality of life in many ways. For instance, developing adequate strength enables us to perform daily functions or participate in recreational sports more easily and comfortably. For an elderly man, adequate strength may mean the ability to shovel snow or tend to his garden. For the competitive athlete, strength may supply the winning edge needed for success.

In addition to allowing one to perform daily tasks more efficiently, increased muscle mass will protect the joints and thus will help prevent debilitating wear-and-tear injuries such as tendinitis and arthritis. Strength also may lessen the severity of injury, says Brittenham, because the bony surfaces of areas such as the knee are better protected and thus able to withstand more trauma.

"The better the musculature is developed, the more coordination and agility you will have," adds Brittenham, who also serves as the strength and conditioning coach for the Indianapolis Pacers professional basketball team. "Thus you have better tools to withstand a fall or to react to a potential injury situation."

For instance, a well-developed trunk and torso will help prevent the most common ailment in society -- low-back pain.

"This is one of the key areas we concentrate on in our strength training programs," says Brittenham. About 70% of all people with sedentary jobs will suffer low-back pain, he adds.

Flexibility of the lower back and other areas will improve with strength training "if the muscles are exercised through the full range of motion," says Semenick. "For a long time people have associated inflexibility with weight lifters. However, the fact is weight lifters are much more flexible than the general population."

Studies have demonstrated that physical activity will increase bone mineral content, and weight-bearing exercise has been associated with greater bone density. Sports medicine experts agree that it's reasonable to conclude that strength training is beneficial in the prevention of osteoporosis, a condition -- largely affecting postmenopausal women -- in which bone mass decreases and leads to fractures.

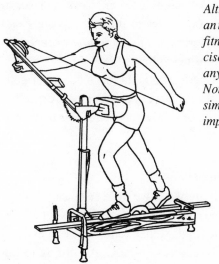

Although strength training is an important part of a balanced fitness program, aerobic exercise should be the foundation of any exercise program. The NordicTrack cross-country ski simulator is an excellent way to improve cardiovascular health.

Strength training is generally regarded as an anaerobic activity, but it may elicit some of the health gain associated with aerobic exercise. Circuit weight training, which is a series of weight training repetitions for about 30 minutes at a rapid pace, may yield some small aerobic gains, according to studies. And some researchers suggest that circuit training may help stimulate high-density lipoprotein cholesterol (HDL-C), the so-called good cholesterol. But experts agree that 25 minutes a day on a cross-country ski machine is a far better way to improve aerobic capacity and blood lipids.

Looking Good, Feeling Good

The sense of well-being created from strength training may yield physiological benefits that far outweigh the physical benefits. For instance, improved appearance derived from strength work may do wonders for one's self-confidence in work and social settings. A strong physique contributes to improved posture and generally creates a positive impression among fellow workers and prospective employers and business clients.

"About 80% of the American population has a poor self-image," says Brittenham. "That poor image can adversely affect many careers and families, and certainly may contribute to depression and emotional problems."

Physiological Adaptations

What happens to the body when we do resistance training? Muscles hypertrophy, or they increase in size. They get larger, stronger, and more resilient. On the other hand, when a person is inactive, muscles atrophy, or decrease in size. According to Semenick, strength training experts agree that the main physiological change caused by strength training is an increase in the size of the muscle fibers, not an increase in the number of fibers. However, some animal studies suggest that hyperplasia -- the increase in muscle fibers -- does occur to some extent.

"Strength training tends to selectively hypertrophy the fast-twitch muscle fibers (the stronger, faster contracting fibers useful in forceful movements)," says Semenick. "Weight training doesn't have much of an effect on the slow-twitch fibers. Building slow-twitch fiber is best left to aerobic training."

For example, the strongest individuals have predominantly fast-twitch fiber, while long-distance runners have more slow-twitch fibers. Studies of power lifters and bodybuilders found that different training regimens may affect the type of muscle fiber that grows. For instance, power lifters, who train largely with low volume and heavy loads, will have a greater ratio of fast-twitch to slow-twitch fiber area than bodybuilders, whose training consists largely of higher volume and lighter loads.

Hypertrophy is controlled in part by the amount of testosterone in the body. Because women generally have less of this male hormone than men, it's difficult for women who train similarly to men to match the increases in muscle mass achieved in those men. Also, the sudden increase in muscle strength in males during puberty is related to their testosterone increases.

Getting Started

When and how should one go about starting a strength training program? According to Semenick, virtually anyone can begin a program. Prepubescents will experience limited strength gains, but supervised strength training is recommended for them as long as "they exhibit good technique, avoid maximum lifts, and do lots of repetitions with light loads. It's good to start kids early because they learn neuromuscular patterns and techniques, so when they reach puberty they're ahead of the game."

The key for any beginning strength trainer is to proceed cautiously. Semenick suggests that exercisers over the age of 40 or anyone with a preexisting medical condition, such as high blood pressure or a musculoskeletal disorder, should receive their physician's clearance before beginning an exercise program. You should then seek the advice of an exercise specialist who can help you identify strength training goals and chart a program for attaining those goals. This professional should be familiar with the types of exercise modalities that you'll be using and be able to suggest proper warm-up and cool-down exercises. A good coach will review proper technique -- both lifting and breathing -- before allowing you to continue a strength training program alone.

"I generally suggest that the person pick a series of exercises -- usually 8 to 10 -- that will begin working the largest muscle masses of the body and progress to the smallest," says Semenick. "For instance, we would pick four exercises for the lower body and four for the upper body. And then we'd find out what weight the person can handle through the full range of motion in good form for 10 repetitions of each exercise. So if we're working on the Universal weight training machine, we might start with a lineup of leg

---

DeLorme Training Method . . .

Three sets* of each exercise performed at varying degrees of your 10-repetition maximum as follows:

- **First Set:** 50% of RM
  - **Second Set:** 75% of RM
    - **Third Set:** 100% of RM

(Each set = 10-12 reps)

press (lower body), bench press (upper body), leg extensions, lat pull down, hamstring curls, military press, calf raisers, and bicep curls, followed by some abdominal work. Never exhaust the abdominals before a workout."

Semenick recommends that beginners start with the De-Lorme method, which includes three sets of each exercise performed at 50% of your 10-repetition maximum (RM) through the first set; 75% of 10-RM for the second set, and 100% of 10-RM for the third set. So if your 10-RM is 100 pounds on the leg press, you would start with 50 pounds the first set and progress to 75 and 100 pounds on the second and third sets. "The DeLorme system provides a reasonable program that guards against injury," he says, And it's got a built-in warm-up session."

Training should be done at least twice a week but preferably three or four times weekly to adequately stimulate muscle and achieve gains, says Brittenham. Knowing the rest/recovery cycle, in which the muscles adapt to the overload, is critical to the success of the training regimen, he adds. "You should start cautiously; underwork the muscles before you overwork them," he says. " I suggest dividing the body into parts: Work two parts on Monday and Thursday, and work two other parts Tuesday and Friday. Always record your workouts and allow at least one or two days recovery time before reworking a muscle group. Small microscopic tears may occur in muscle fibers, particularly at the onset of a strength training program, so they may need a little more time to recover. However, with time the muscles will adapt. The key is listening to your body. Performing good warm-up and cool-down exercises will also help eliminate soreness."

Dangers of Strength Training

The biggest fault of many beginning weight trainers is starting too fast, too heavy, and too early. "The biggest mistake of strength trainers is compromising technique for resistance," says Sol Brandys, director of exercise and conditioning for the Northwest Racquet, Swim and Health Clubs in Minneapolis and St. Paul. "Weight training is a macho thing for so many people. They want to move as much weight as possible, and they don't care if they do it properly. They like to take shortcuts. Instead of putting in the time necessary to achieve their goals, they find ways to reduce the time and effort of their investment. The result is usually injury and postponement of one's goals."

Ignoring proper breathing techniques is another risk. If strength trainers use the Valsalva maneuver -- holding one's breath on the effort part of the exercise -- blood pressure may increase to dangerously high levels and lightheadedness may result. "People must learn to exhale slowly on the difficult part of exercises," Semenick says. "It's hard to breathe normally, especially during maximum lifts."

Exercise for a Lifetime

The key to reasonable strength training is to design a program that you can perform for a lifetime. Lean muscle mass is the critical factor, says Brittenham, and to develop and maintain muscle mass and tone, you can't leave muscles unattended. "To keep functioning at peak performance it's essential that we keep exercising," he says. "Strength training is a vital component of a balanced fitness program."

Strength Training Has Come Out of the Locker Room

Steven J. Fleck, Ph.D.

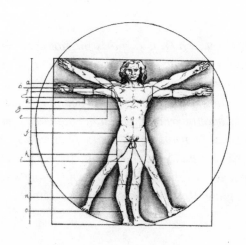

*❝ Strength training is no longer the ❞
exclusive domain of elite
athletes. Rather, the potential
health and quality of life benefits
will be the focus of all
comprehensive fitness programs
of the future.*

Steven J. Fleck, Ph.D. *is a sports physiologist with the
United States Olympic Committee whose major area is
strength/power and anaerobic training. He has designed
resistance training programs for the health enthusiast as
well as national/international caliber athletes and pre-
sented resistance training seminars in the U.S., South
America, Europe and South East Asia. He has written numerous articles on resistance training and co-authored the
book,* Designing Resistance Training Programs.

6

During the 1970's and 80's "aerobics" was the battle cry of the fitness craze. And indeed, aerobic or endurance training does result in increased cardiovascular fitness and its associated health benefits. However, cardiovascular fitness alone should not be understood to mean "balanced" or "total fitness." You've probably known a person who ran, swam or cycled religiously but who lacked the flexibility to bend over and touch their toes or the upper body strength to carry their luggage through the airport. Aerobic exercise is great for increasing cardiovascular fitness but it does not necessarily lead to increased flexibility, strength, or power.

"Balanced fitness" refers to a combination of cardiovascular, flexibility and strength training exercises that provide the health and quality of life benefits of all three. Strength training is no longer the exclusive domain of elite athletes. Rather, the potential health and quality of life benefits will be the focus of all comprehensive fitness programs of the future.

One aspect of strength training that has been misunderstood is the effect it has on cardiovascular fitness and the risk factors of cardiovascular disease. Many people believe that strength training increases resting heart rate and blood pressure, while in fact, scientific studies report either no change or a slight but significant decrease in both resting heart rate and blood pressure. Decreased resting heart rate and blood pressure may be associated with strength training programs which utilize large volumes (total number of pounds lifted). These programs normally use moderate resistance and high numbers of repetitions (10 to 15) per exercise, multiple sets of each exercise, and short rest periods between exercises (less than 1 minute). Hypertension (resting high blood pressure) when found in elite resistance trained athletes may be associated with androgen use, very large increases in muscle mass, chronic overtraining, and essential hypertension.

Another positive adaptation normally associated with cardiovascular training programs is increased peak oxygen consumption (VO2 peak). Normal and higher than normal peak oxygen consumptions have been reported in elite resistance trained athletes (body builders, Olympic lifters, power lifters). Short term (8 - 20 weeks) training studies on average individuals demonstrate that resistance training can cause increases in peak oxygen consumption of approximately 5 percent in both men and women. As with resting heart rate and blood pressure, increases in peak oxygen consumption appear to be associated with programs using a high volume of training. However, these modest increases in peak oxygen consumption are much smaller than the 15 to 20 percent increases normally associated with running, swimming, cycling or other cardiovascular programs of the same duration. Thus, to achieve balanced fitness it is important to perform some type of cardiovascular training in addition to strength training.

The effect strength training has upon the blood lipid profile, one cardiovascular risk factor, is still controversial. Decreased total cholesterol, decreased low density lipoprotein (LDL) and increased high density lipoprotein (HDL) are positive adaptations to many cardiovascular training programs. Research on strength training, on the other hand, has failed to provide definitive results. Some studies indicate positive adaptations to strength training while others report no changes in these blood parameters. It should be noted, however, that some of these studies have been criticized for limitations in their design. (These criticisms have centered upon such things as small number of subjects, no control of diet and taking only one blood sample from each subject.) It does appear, however, that resistance training can have a positive effect on the lipid profile and that it does <u>not</u> have a negative impact. This lack of definitive results regarding the effect strength training has on the lipid profile is another reason why cardiovascular training must be included in a balanced fitness program.

One of the most visible and positive changes unique to strength training is increased muscle strength. Besides the satisfaction of putting another five or ten pounds on your bench press, there are many health and quality of life related benefits to increased strength. First, greater muscle strength makes many daily activities easier -- lifting a child, carrying the groceries up a flight of stairs -- easier and more comfortable. In addition, increased upper body strength will improve performance in many recreational activities

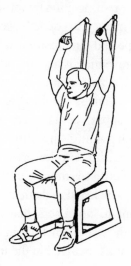

Many daily activities can be made easier with increased upper body strength.

such as putting a little more power in your tennis serves or golf shots. This can be especially important to women, who are generally only about 50 percent as strong as men in the upper body.

Another benefit of strength training is aesthetics and the improved self-image associated with a well defined body. Many people who start a strength training program are concerned that they'll "bulk up" or gain body weight. This is especially true of women. The vast majority of studies indicate that the strength training program the average man or women has the time or desire to perform will cause no increase in total body weight. This is because any increase in muscle tissue is balanced by a corresponding loss of fat resulting in no net gain in body weight. Greater muscle mass accompanied by a loss of fat is also the reason for the slim arm and leg measurements reported in many studies. These results are in sharp contrast to many peoples' image of strength training which has been created by body builders and other athletes who strength train to build muscle mass. The people who achieve these results have a genetic predisposition for muscle hypertrophy and their bulk is the result of many years of daily work. Most people who strength train will shape and tone their muscles but add very little bulk.

Injury prevention is another possible result of strength training. The incidence of injuries caused by overuse such as "tennis elbow" and "swimmers shoulder" is lower in athletes who strength train on a regular basis compared to athletes who don't perform any type of strength training. In addition, the reoccurrence of these injuries is less frequent. This lowered incidence of injury is probably related to the increased strength and power of the muscles, tendons and ligaments which makes them more capable of tolerating stress. It is important to note here that these, like most adaptations associated with a strength training program, occur only in the muscles and joints involved in the training program.

One of the most common complaints among both athletes and

non-athletes is lower back pain. In many instances the pain is associated with weak abdominal musculature and "tight" hamstrings and can be greatly reduced or alleviated completely by a training program designed to strengthen the abdominal muscles and in-

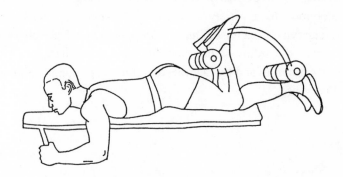

Strengthening the abdominal muscles and increasing the flexibility of the hamstrings can greatly reduce or alleviate lower back pain.

crease the flexibility of the hamstring muscle group. This type of conservative treatment of lower back pain clearly demonstrates the need for "balanced fitness."

One of the less visible adaptations to resistance training is increased bone mass. In humans it has been shown that physical activity including resistance training can increase bone mass. It appears that bone mass is increased when the bones are engaged in a load bearing activity or when forceful contractions take place in the muscles responsible for moving a particular joint and the associated bones. Thus it may be possible with resistance training not only to increase bone mass in the legs and axial skeleton but also in the arms. As the human life span increases, osteoporosis becomes more of a concern (especially in women) because total bone mass decreases with age. This loss of bone mass leads to the increased possibility of fractures in old age. Resistance training's ability to increase bone mass in the lower as well as the upper body could have long lasting health benefits.

Potentially, almost any form of exercise or physical activity can have a positive effect on balanced fitness. Some of these effects are common to a variety of activities, others are unique to a particular type of exercise. Thus it is important to balance all forms of exercise -- cardiovascular, flexibility and strength training -- in a fitness program and by that means achieve optimum health and quality of life.

The Value of
Strength Training

Ellen Hillegass, MMSc, PT, CCS

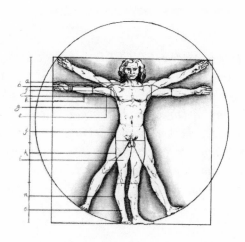

"   *The importance of strength*   *"*
training can no longer be
ignored. It provides a wide
variety of health and occupa-
tional benefits essential to quality
of life. Combined with aerobic
exercise, it creates what is now
referred to as 'balanced fitness.'

Ellen Hillegass, MMSc, PT, CCS is an American Physical
Therapy Association (APTA) board certified cardiopul-
monary clinical specialist. She is currently the Cardiopul-
monary Program Director at Georgia State University
and is a fellow of the American Association of Cardiovas-
cular and Pulmonary Rehabilitation. She has extensive ex-
perience teaching fitness and fitness evaluation in continu-
ing education courses throughout the United States.

7

Strength training has long been considered the poor cousin to aerobics. Its sole purpose has been to build strength and muscle in brawny young men. Only within the last couple of years has the medical profession begun to examine the many positive aspects of strength training.

Traditionally, strength training has been performed to change or improve one's physical appearance and/or to compete in strength or power lifting competitions. When strength training <u>was</u> researched for its effects beyond improved muscle mass and strength, indications of elevated blood pressure and cholesterol were discovered. Strength training became misrepresented from these negative findings, and unfortunately, these negative findings did not distinguish the factors that directly affected blood pressure, such as muscle groups worked, lifting style, and the amount of resistance used.

In contrast, aerobic exercise has been positively received by both the medical community and the public, and has become closely associated with fitness and health. Numerous research studies have shown that continuous submaximal aerobic exercise, done regularly for 20 minutes or more, decreases the risk of heart disease by improving aerobic capacity, decreasing body fat, improving cholesterol levels and decreasing stress. Individuals who perform regular aerobic exercise also have improved endurance in occupational and recreational activities, improved self-esteem, and better productivity on the job.

Balanced Fitness

In recent years, however, the medical community has begun to reconsider their understanding of the value of strength training. This is evident in the revised exercise guidelines released in May by the American College of Sports Medicine, which include a recommendation for "strength training of moderate intensity at a minimum of two times per week." These new recommendations are in no way intended to detract from the importance of aerobic exercise, as aerobic exercise with all its benefits remains the essential component of health and fitness. But the importance of strength training can no longer be ignored. It provides a wide variety of health and occupational benefits essential to quality of life. Combined with aerobic exercise, it creates what is now referred to as "balanced fitness."

"Strength Training," What Is It?

Strength training is defined as any form of exercise which systematically overloads a muscle or muscles to improve the contractile activity. The intensity and progressive nature of the overload helps determine the amount and type of strength gained. Muscles perform a wide variety of functions that range from static activity to high velocity activity. Therefore strength training can be performed using a variety of methods depending upon the result desired. Body builders and power lifters, for example, perform exercises which develop muscle mass in order to increase the weight they can lift and/or enhance their physiques. On the other hand, sprinters and other athletes who require speed perform exercises which develop endurance and speed in the desired muscle activity.

The three methods most commonly used to elicit muscle contraction are *isometric, isotonic* and *isokinetic.* When a muscle exerts force, but does not change in length, it is said to contract *isometrically.* In other words, the force exerted by the muscle is equal to the force exerted by the resistance, and no movement occurs. Isometric contractions are important for stabilizing movements and for maintaining given joint positions. This method of training is frequently used to strengthen extremely weak muscles that cannot generate a force great enough to overcome the weight of the bone to be moved. One example of this type of training is the practice of squeezing a rubber ball to increase strength in the forearm. Isometric exercise is also utilized when treating arthritic extremities when movement of the joint is not desirable, and with post injury and post operative populations.

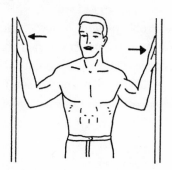

An isometric exercise is one in which the force exerted by the muscle is equal to the force exerted by the resistance, and no movement occurs.

Pain and swelling, as well as further joint damage, is prevented with this method of strength training. This type of training traditionally will not increase muscle bulk or muscular endurance, but will improve strength and thereby improve function.

Isotonic training is the more traditional method of strength training, typified by the use of free weights, barbells and weight machines such as the Nautilus and the Universal Gym. These systems load the muscles in one of two ways: the constant load method and the variable resistance method. Free weights, barbells and many weight machines offer a constant load to the muscle, whereas other weight machines such as cam-type machines vary the resistance throughout the range of motion. The primary advantages of isotonic training are the availability of equipment and the fact that active contraction results in lengthening (eccentric muscle contraction) or shortening (concentric muscle contraction) of the muscle fiber as tension develops to overcome resistance.

Controversy continues over the results of various isotonic strength training methods. At the two extremes are high resistance training (high weight) with low repetitions, and low resistance training (low weight) with high repetitions. Studies indicate that high resistance, low repetition training will increase muscle mass, but will not improve endurance, whereas low resistance, high repetition training will improve endurance and strength but will not increase muscle mass.

Problems with isotonic training include the inability to develop muscle speed, the fact that it loads the muscle with the resistance at the weakest point (which may not be safe), and trauma, usually identified by muscle soreness the day following an exercise session.

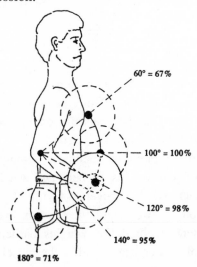

60° = 67%

100° = 100%

120° = 98%

140° = 95%

180° = 71%

Because muscles have weak and strong points throughout the range of motion, the muscle will be worked differently at different points in the range of motion. In this example, the bicep muscle is weakest at the 100 degree point and therefore is working at 100% of its maximum. At higher and lower points it's easier for the muscle to lift the weight and therefore the bicep doesn't work at its maximum capacity.

Isokinetic (accommodating resistance) training has become the preferred method of strength training in recent years. Training the muscles isokinetically means that the speed of the lever arm is proportional to resistance throughout the range of motion. In other words, resistance is in direct proportion to the force offered. Therefore, greater force results in greater resistance. This type of training has been found to be highly functional, especially in developing muscular endurance.

The disadvantages of isokinetic machines has always been price, since typically they could provide only one training modality per unit. But today, with moderately priced equipment such as the Nordic Fitness Chair manufactured by NordicTrack, this is no longer a problem. The Nordic Fitness Chair, designed for in-home use, eliminates the complexity of other strength training programs, and allows for up to 20 different exercises that increase upper body strength.

The Nordic Fitness Chair eliminates the complexity of most other strength training programs.

Why Strength Train?

Strength training provides functional and health benefits to people of almost every population. From improving a basketball player's vertical jump to increasing the force behind the baseball bat, athletes of all varieties use strength training to improve their performance. That strength is just as important to the non-athlete. Picking up a child, carrying the groceries, and opening a jar of peanut butter are all daily activities which can be made easier and more comfortable with greater muscle strength.

Recently, strength training has been associated with improvements in muscle endurance in addition to strength gains. One particular study measured endurance in terms of the number of repetitions a person was able to perform before exhaustion. After eight weeks of training, endurance capacity, as measured by the number of repetitions the person was able to perform, had increased. What this means in terms of lifestyle benefits is the ability to weed the garden, rake the lawn, and run down the concourse with a heavy briefcase.

The muscles of the body have often been compared to the shock absorbers of a car. They absorb the shock and pounding the body takes in simply performing daily activities, and strong muscles do the job more effectively. They help protect ligaments, tendons, bones, and joint capsules from the pounding they take by simply running for a bus. Performing strength training exercises, then, can help protect the body from injury.

Health Benefits of Strength Training

Cardiovascular fitness, improved cholesterol profiles, and a lower incidence of heart disease and hypertension are all health benefits commonly associated with aerobic exercise. Indeed, strength training in the past has been associated with a higher risk of hypertension and heart disease. However, in reevaluating the data, it was discovered that many of these early studies utilized professional athletes working with extremely high weight and few repetitions and that, at least in some instances, the athletes were using steroids to enhance muscle mass and performance. Newer studies report that in strength training programs utilizing lower weights and higher repetitions, there is a tendency towards decreases in LDL (bad) cholesterol, increases in HDL (good) cholesterol, and decreases in diastolic blood pressure.

In fact, the medical community is so convinced of the importance of strength training in improving and maintaining an individual's functional ability and self image, many cardiopulmonary rehabilitation programs are adding strength training to their fitness routines. This is in contrast with the tradition of prescribing only aerobic exercises in rehabilitation applications. For the most part, these programs prescribe low resistance, high repetition training modales.

Occupational therapy is another application which utilizes strength training extensively. Typically, the goal of these programs is to return individuals to their work place capable of performing their tasks following a muscoskeletal injury. This usually involves rehabilitation by traditional therapeutic modalities. Strength training exercises involving job-specific movements are then incorporated to increase muscle strength and endurance. Both resistance and repetitions are progressively increased over a period of weeks or months until the individual is able to perform the task effectively through an eight hour shift.

Strength training should not be perceived as an exercise intended solely for developing the physique. No, strength training now has a definite place in maintaining both health and quality of life in every population. It increases the individual's ability to perform daily, recreational and occupational activities. And it enhances health by protecting the body, increasing endurance and helping to develop and maintain cardiovascular fitness. But strength training alone is only a component. It must be performed in combination with aerobic exercise and an appropriate diet to achieve balanced fitness and thus, improve health and quality of life.

Strength Training Guidelines During Pregnancy

Susan Johnson, Ed.D.

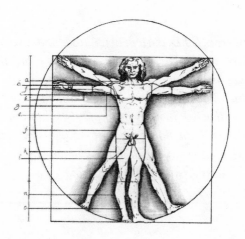

" *An individualized, closely* *"*
monitored exercise program can
help prepare the woman for the
hard work of pregnancy, delivery,
and care of the newborn.

Susan Johnson, Ed.D. *is a teacher, author and researcher, and is currently the Director of Continuing Education at the Institute for Aerobics Research in Dallas, Texas. Her public education background is at both the teaching and supervisory levels. She has been published in numerous trade journals in the dance and fitness industry, and has been recognized as an outstanding educator by the Aerobics and Fitness Association of America.*

8

Pregnancy & Exercise

Pregnancy, delivery, and care for a newborn is hard work. That hard work is easier and safer for both mother and baby if the mother is physically fit. And while current research offers no conclusive evidence to support the popular notion that regular exercise will change the length or quality of labor and delivery, decrease fetal or maternal complications or improve the health of the child, most studies show that safe, moderate exercise has no or minimal negative effects on the expectant mother with no medical complications.

As reported in *New Aerobics for Women*, by Dr. Kenneth Cooper and his wife Millie Cooper, experience at the Aerobics Center indicates that women who exercise throughout their pregnancies report:

1) fewer Caesarean section deliveries;
2) facilitated labor;
3) reduced recovery time;
4) weight gain within the optimum range;
5) better control of body fat;
6) reduced constipation;
7) better sleep;
8) increased ability to cope with physical and emotional stresses of pregnancy;

9)   increased energy;

10) protection against back pain from postural shift; and

11) improved postpartum muscle tone.

In addition, prenatal and postpartum exercisers report psychological benefits such as improved mood, higher self-esteem and simply looking and feeling better.

    While there is no medical consensus indicating that healthy pregnant women should avoid exercise, most experts suggest a conservative approach. Definitive guidelines have not been determined because of the ethical ramifications of testing for maternal and fetal health and safety at the upper levels of intense exercise. Most current recommendations, including the ones presented in this article, are based on common sense, current thinking among respected experts, available research on animals and humans, and the desire to promote the greatest physical fitness within the parameters of maximum safety for mother and fetus.

Designing An Exercise Program

    An exercise program for pregnant women should meet four basic criteria. First, and most importantly, it must be safe. Because of the radical changes that occur during pregnancy, the exercise program must be designed to insure maternal and fetal safety. Second, the program should be enjoyable. If the individual does not enjoy the activity or exercise, she is more likely to drop out of the program. Third, the program should be effective. The activities or exercises should be long enough, hard enough, and frequent enough to insure that conditioning occurs. Again, a cautious, low-risk approach is recommended until research provides more definite exercise guidelines. This means that frequency, intensity and duration of activities may need to be gradually reduced, especially as pregnancy progresses into the last trimester. Finally, the exercise program should be balanced to include aerobics, flexibility, and strength work. The importance of muscle strength and endurance as part of a balanced program to develop total fitness is often overlooked. Many prenatal and postpartum exercise programs address only aerobic activities such as walking or swimming. Therefore, strength training considerations and guidelines will be the major focus of this article.

Balanced Fitness: One Component of a Healthy Pregnancy

The major benefits of exercise to a pregnant woman include maintaining muscle tone, strength and endurance; protecting against back pain; feeling energetic; and enhancing mood and self-image. These benefits can be appreciated during both the prenatal and postpartum periods if precautions and safety guidelines are followed under the supervision of a physician. An individualized, closely monitored exercise program can help prepare the woman for the hard work of pregnancy, delivery, and care of the newborn.

Although this article emphasizes the importance of strength training, it is important that a pregnant women participate in a program of "balanced fitness" which includes aerobic, flexibility, and strength work. It must also be remembered that exercise is just one part of a healthy lifestyle during pregnancy. Regular prenatal care, good nutrition, adequate rest, avoidance of tobacco, alcohol and unnecessary drugs are just as important. There are many choices that the mother can make to positively influence her own health and that of her developing child.

Strength Training

Essentially, there are two kinds of strength: 1) muscular strength, often called absolute strength and 2) muscular endurance, often called dynamic strength. Absolute strength refers to the ability to generate the maximum amount of force in a single muscular contraction. For example, if on an initial test an individual bench presses 80 pounds and on a later test she is able to lift 120, then her absolute strength has improved. Dynamic strength refers to the ability to generate force for repeated muscular contractions without undue fatigue. For example, if on an initial test an individual performs 20 sit-ups in a minute and on a later test she is able to perform 40 sit-ups, then her dynamic strength has improved.

If a muscle is regularly exercised by contracting against resistance, it will accommodate this demand by growing stronger and larger. This is called hypertrophy. If the resistance is low to moderate and the contractions are repeated several times, the person will be more likely to develop dynamic strength or muscle endurance. If the resistance is high or very high and the contractions are repeated only a few times, then the person will be more likely to develop absolute strength or muscular strength. It is interesting to note that because of different hormones and number of muscle fibers, men will tend to "bulk up" with strength training whereas women will tend to tone and define their muscles.

Although differing opinions have been expressed, the general consensus among medical authorities is that properly conducted strength training programs are safe for healthy pregnant women. According to "Women and Exercise," *ACOG Technical Bulletin*, 1985, published by the American College of Obstetricians and Gynecologists, "Regardless of prior exercise habits and level of fitness, most healthy pregnant women without medical or obstetric complications can lift weights safely and beneficially." Among the many possible benefits of strength training are: good posture, prevention of low back pain, strengthening of the pelvic floor, and prevention of diastasis recti (separation of the abdominal muscles).

Some medical authorities have suggested that pregnancy is an inappropriate time to begin a new, vigorous exercise regimen or to intensify the training effort. The previously sedentary expectant mother should engage in exercise forms that maintain or slightly improve current fitness levels. In other words, she should participate in low levels of exercise which progress slowly. The previously fit expectant mother can continue her exercise program but should decrease the frequency, intensity, and/or duration of training if she is accustomed to working out at rigorous intensities. Both sedentary and fit individuals entering motherhood should avoid exercising to exhaustion during the first trimester when fetal attachment and early development occurs. The optimal time to cautiously increase exercise quality and quantity is during the second trimester when both the risks associated with exercise and the discomforts of pregnancy are minimal. It is inadvisable to increase exercise quality and quantity during the third trimester when there is increased potential for musculoskeletal and physiological injury to mother and fetus.

Safety and Medical Considerations

The importance of working closely with a physician when exercising during pregnancy cannot be overemphasized. Prenatal and postpartum exercise programs must be designed for the unique conditions of the particular individual as she progresses through the various stages of pregnancy. What may have been appropriate prior to or during one stage of pregnancy may no longer be applicable. There is a great deal of variability in the way different women respond to pregnancy, and the exercise prescription should be personalized on a case by case basis. The physician needs to evaluate each person with respect to prior and current health and fitness status, medical limitations, physical and physiological changes, and medical history during previous pregnancies.

Once an individual has been cleared for exercise, she must be taught to recognize the warning signs and symptoms which may alert her to a potential problem. The following "red flags" should signal the person to stop exercising and contact her physician. Some of these may be normal reactions to advancing pregnancy, but it is prudent to discuss the occurrence of any signs with a physician.

Warning Signs:

- pain, especially abdominal or chest
- dizziness or faintness
- excessive shortness of breath
- excessive fatigue
- difficulty walking
- sudden swelling of ankles, hands, or face
- insufficient weight gain (less than 1 kg/month during last two trimesters)
- swelling, pain, and redness in calf of one leg (phlebitis)
- bleeding from the vagina
- increased blood pressure
- back or pubic pain
- any "gush" of vaginal fluid
- absence of fetal movement
- persistent, severe headaches and/or visual disturbance
- persistent contractions (more than 6-8/hour) which may suggest the onset of labor

A pregnant woman is neither fragile nor incapacitated, but she is physically different from a non-pregnant woman. The physical and physiological changes she undergoes may make her more vulnerable to injury when she exercises, and there are potential hazards for the fetus, as well. Following are the major changes that require exercise modification in a prenatal and postpartum strength training program.

Physical and Physiological Changes During Pregnancy

Resting heart rate. During pregnancy, maternal blood volume increases by 30 percent or more, elevating cardiac output. Because of this increase, the heart rate during exercise may rise much higher and quicker than that of a non-pregnant exerciser. Using a perceived exertion scale during strength training as a means of comparison to the non-pregnant state may be a good way to monitor exercise intensity and maintain a level of exertion not higher than before pregnancy.

Blood flow. During exercise, blood is shunted away from the internal organs including the uterus and placenta and toward the working muscles. The greater and more prolonged the muscular work, the more blood is diverted. Since exercise guidelines at higher intensities have yet to be defined, a safe recommendation for strength training during pregnancy is to work at moderate intensities and to rest briefly between exercise sets. The Valsalva maneuver should be avoided since this is hypothesized to cause diversion of blood flow from the internal organs to the muscles. (The Valsalva maneuver occurs when a person holds her breath and closes the glottis in the throat while lifting weights. This can be avoided by breathing out during muscular exertion.)

Hormones. The joints of the body are less stable during pregnancy making the woman more susceptible to injury. Hormones such as estrogen, progesterone, and elastin make a pregnant woman's connective tissues, such as ligaments, more lax not only in the pelvis but in the ankles, feet, hips, knees, and shoulders. After giving birth, it takes 6 to 16 weeks for hormone levels to return to normal. Because of these softer tissues and unstable joints, lighter resistance with more repetitions is recommended.

Most experts will agree that lighter resistances such as three to five pound dumbbells will probably pose no problem to the pregnant woman. Some have even suggested that "heavier" resistances can be used safely, but no guidelines have been established for "how heavy." Current research studies investigating strength training during pregnancy did not exceed 50% 1RM (one repetition max) or about one half the weight a person can lift one time. Beginning exercisers should work out with less weight than already conditioned people and both should try to maintain or gently improve strength rather than embark on a vigorous muscle-building campaign.

In general, because of joint laxity, pregnant women should avoid positions which may excessively flex or extend ligaments and tendons such as deep squats and knee bends.

Adrenal hormones. Epinephrine and norepinephrine levels increase during exercise. Norepinephrine has the potential for precipitating premature labor in susceptible individuals. While a mild increase in uterine activity following exercise is common, a physician should be consulted if there is pelvic pressure or regular patterns of contractions.

Body temperature. Basal body temperature is higher during pregnancy and it is hypothesized that the temperature response may be further exaggerated during exercise. Animal studies indicate that increased temperature may cause abnormalities in the development of the fetus. The problem of hyperthermia or overheating is of special concern because the fetus has no mechanisms such as perspiration or respiration to dissipate excess heat. In general, pregnant women should not exercise in hot and humid weather, when they have a fever, or when they feel overheated. Indoor exercise during especially hot and humid weather may be the ideal alternative. Dehydration can also increase core temperatures to dangerous levels, and pregnant exercisers should drink liquids before, during, and after exercise as necessary to replenish body fluids.

Enlarged uterus and the supine position. Pregnant women should not lie on their backs to exercise after the fourth month of pregnancy since the enlarged uterus may block the flow of blood through the vena cava which carries blood back to the heart, and can potentially interfere with blood flow to the placenta.

Enlarged uterus and the lower back. As the uterus enlarges, the trunk tends to pull forward. To compensate, the individual brings her shoulders back. This posture is called lordosis or "swayback." The arched position places stress on the back and hips resulting commonly in lower back pain. Exercises which use the arched or hyperextended position should be avoided. The pelvic tilt exercise performed in the standing, sitting, side-lying, or all-fours position can help counter the tendency toward lordosis. The exercise is performed by contracting the buttocks and abdomen while gently rotating the pubic bone forward and upward and holding the position for 10 seconds.

To further protect the lower back, avoid the forward flexed position as in bending over with straight legs to pick up weights. This position combined with the extra body weight of pregnancy places excessive stress on several structures of the lower back including the intervertebral discs.

Enlarged uterus and balance. A pregnant woman's enlarged uterus and breasts raises her center of gravity. This influences the sense of balance and makes walking more difficult and ordinary movements somewhat more awkward. Strength training positions should therefore employ stable bases of support and good body alignment. Shoes should be selected which offer stability and support to minimize the risk of tripping.

Enlarged uterus and respiration. During the third trimester of pregnancy, the enlarged uterus will push the diaphragm upward causing the person to feel uncomfortable and often short of breath. This is a signal to cut back further on the intensity of exercise.

Nutrition. Approximately 300 extra calories are needed daily to meet the metabolic requirements of pregnancy. Women who are actively exercising should consume additional calories to accommodate the energy expenditure of the exercise. For example, if a woman expends 200 to 300 calories during her workout, she should add approximately the same number of extra calories of nutrient-dense food to her diet. This is important because glucose levels are generally lower in pregnant women. Also, they use carbohydrates at a greater rate during exercise increasing the risk of hypoglycemia (low blood sugar) after prolonged or strenuous exercise periods. To insure mother and fetus receive the proper nutrients, dietary restriction and exercise for weight loss should be reserved for after the birth of the baby. However, women who breast feed should maintain five to ten pounds over their pre-pregnancy weight (if they were not overweight to begin with) to support the energy demands of lactation. Generally, breast feeding requires up to 500 extra calories per day.

Pelvic floor. The physical and hormonal changes of pregnancy cause stretching and laxity in the supporting tissues of the pelvis. Vaginal delivery causes further stretching. Kegel exercises, which help tone the muscles of the pelvic floor can be performed during pregnancy and again soon after the birth. These exercises can be done by stopping and starting the flow of urine.

Healing after delivery. Healing time varies from woman to woman but usually takes six weeks to three months. The site where the placenta was attached to the uterus needs time to mend as do tears, episiotomies, or incisions from Caesarian section deliveries.

A physically active woman before and during pregnancy will be more ready to resume physical activity after giving birth than a sedentary one, but both should ease gradually into higher levels of activity and consult regularly with their physician.

Physiological Adaptations of Strength Training

Ted Lambrinides, Ph.D.

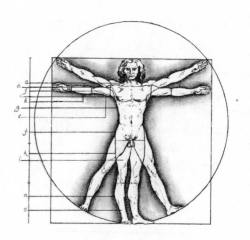

" *Not so long ago, many sports* "
medicine professionals excluded
strength training from any
exercise prescription. However,
in the past 15 to 20 years more
and more research has begun to
shed light on the benefits of
strength training.

Ted Lambrinides *is a graduate of Ohio State University where he did his masters and doctoral work in exercise physiology. He is currently the Director of Research for the Hammer Corporation in Cincinnati, Ohio and a member of the American College of Sports Medicine. He is the former Director of Education for Nautilus Midwest, and is often quoted in articles pertaining to exercise and physical fitness.*

9

Not so long ago, many sports medicine professionals excluded strength training from any exercise prescription. The sport was viewed as the exclusive domain of sweaty men with outsized biceps. However, in the past 15 to 20 years more and more research has begun to shed light on the physiological and psychological benefits of strength training. In fact, the American College of Sports Medicine has updated its position paper, "The Recommended Quantity and Quality of Exercise for Developing and Maintaining Fitness in Healthy Adults," to include recommendations on strength training.

Before we look at the physiological benefits of strength training, it should be mentioned that a strength training program needs basically two things: 1) a form of resistance (machines, free weights, rubber bands, etc.) and 2) progression -- as the muscles adapt during strength training one must continually and systematically attempt to overload the muscles for results to continue. Progression can be either more repetitions at a given resistance (compared to a previous workout) or more resistance per repetition (compared to a previous workout).

Strength Adaptations

One of the first adaptations which occurs in the body when a strength training program is begun is in the nervous system. During the first 4 to 6 weeks of a strength training program, most trainees will experience rapid improvements in strength. Most of this initial strength gain can be attributed to a reduction in neural inhibitions. In other words, the body is able to recruit a greater number of muscle fibers while training.

After these initial improvements in the nervous system, strength gained can be directly attributed to improvements in muscle hypertrophy. When a muscle hypertrophies (enlarges), it increases the amount of contractive proteins (actin and myosin) in individual muscle fibers. Most research pertaining to muscle hypertrophy indicates that the size of existing muscle fibers increases, not the number of muscle fibers.

Did you know?

- The human body has over 600 muscles containing more than 6 billion microscopic muscle fibers. Each fiber is so strong that it can support more than 1,000 times its own weight.

- The skeletal muscles make up from 40 to 50 percent of total body weight.

- The production of voluntary movements by skeletal muscle is one of the most essential activities of the body.

- You have approximately the same number of muscle fibers in your body now as when you were an infant. Of course, as you grew from a child to an adult, the fibers grew bigger and stronger, but the total number probably hasn't changed much at all, if any.

The benefits of muscle development go beyond having more strength and an attractive physique. It increases lean body mass. Since the amount of calories one burns is highly correlated to their percentage of lean body mass, a body with a higher percentage of lean mass will expend more calories. And not just while exercising, while driving the car, walking down the street, even sleeping.

For the elderly population, strength training is particularly important. Muscle tissue decreases in the non-active individual, slowing down the metabolic rate and making daily tasks, such as picking up the grandchildren, more difficult.

Strength training provides the strength necessary to continue to perform daily chores and activities, allowing for greater independence which in turn improves self-esteem and quality of life. Dr. William Evans of Tufts University conducted a strength training study on 70 to 80 year old men and found increases in both strength and muscle size.

Along with increases in muscle size and strength, ligaments, tendons and bone become stronger. When a muscle contracts it places enough stress on a bone to slightly bend it, setting up electrical currents that lead to deposition of new bone material. This has tremendous implication for women who have a high risk of developing osteoporosis.

Stronger, more balanced muscles, ligaments, tendons and bone reduce the chance of injury when participating in athletic events or simple day-to-day activities. Further research has shown that in the event of an injury, individuals participating in a strength training program have shorter rehabilitation times than non-strength trained individuals.

Cardiovascular Adaptations

Several studies have shown that strength training can have beneficial effects on blood cholesterol levels. Research by Dr.

Goldberg at the University of Oregon showed that strength training elevated HDL (the good cholesterol) levels and decreased LDL (the bad cholesterol) levels in previously sedentary men and women.

Some types of strength training (competitive Olympic lifting and power lifting) may cause an increase in blood pressure, however this is only a momentary elevation and poses no risk to a healthy individual. Individuals with known cardiovascular conditions can strength train safely provided they follow appropriate training procedures, and work in conjunction with their physician to determine proper exercise guidelines. In fact, research by Harris and Holly found that after nine weeks of a low-resistance, high repetition circuit strength training program for borderline hypertensive individuals, a significant decrease occurred in resting diastolic blood pressure.

In terms of improving cardiovascular endurance, a recent study at Indiana University found that strength training had a significant improvement on running performance.

While strength training can have some positive changes on the cardiovascular system, there are some adaptations which aerobic training can affect to a greater extent. Both strength training and aerobic training complement themselves in an overall training program.

Psychological Benefits

In addition to the physiological effects of strength training, the psychological benefits can be one of the biggest incentives in maintaining a balanced exercise program. Whether one is 18 or 80, developing a stronger body helps create self-confidence and self-esteem, providing a better outlook on life and perhaps better productivity in the workplace and at home.

Strength training has as much to offer the average person as it does the competitive athlete. Incorporating strength training into an existing workout, or beginning a brand-new balanced fitness program is a great way to achieve and maintain health, self-esteem and quality of life.

To Lose Weight,
Add Weight

Beth Livermore

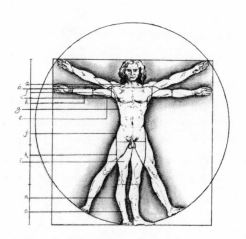

*"   Recently researchers . . . have   "
found that a moderate course of
weight lifting, combined with a
low-fat diet and regular aerobic
exercise, slims people down and
maintains lean body mass more
effectively than any other
combination.*

Beth Livermore *is a freelance writer who has written
various articles on health and fitness, nutrition and the en-
vironment for numerous national magazines. She is a
former Assistant Editor and staff writer for* Health *magazine, and has recently completed a fellowship in science
writing at the Marine Biological Laboratory in Wood-
shole, Mass.*

10

Still dripping from her workout, Judy walked into the examination room. One pinch. Two. This time it was good news. Ten weeks after adding strength training to a routine of careful eating and regular aerobic exercise, she had reduced her body fat from 40 percent to less than 28.5 percent. This represents a loss of 24 pounds of fat. And though she weighed in heavier than her "ideal," she looked and felt better than ever before. "Normally, I'd have to loose another 10 pounds before getting into the clothes I now wear comfortably," she says. "And I have a real healthy glow."

Judy Miller, 56, is just one of a growing number of people who have discovered the merit of pumping iron to subtract fat. Strength training, the discipline of barbells, resistance machines and free weights, has long been associated with the building up of body mass. The most noticed proponents being well muscled men and Amazon women. But recently researchers interested in associated health benefits have found that in addition to preventing bone density loss and amassing strength, a moderate course of weight lifting, combined with a low-fat diet and regular aerobic exercise, slims people down and maintains lean body mass more effectively than any other combination. Strong arming heavy equipment provides a number of psychological benefits, too, say some dieters.

"To be honest, I hated the idea of weight training, so I know why my friends look at me like I'm growing a third ear when I try

to convert them," says Judy. "But I've tried it all, and this works."
The key is in understanding how muscle affects metabolism and
why body composition is more important than body weight.

A Pound of Flesh

"Few people realize it, but most of us loose quite a lot of
muscle when we diet," says Dori Moody, the exercise physiologist
who monitored Judy's progress at The Women's Club Health and
Fitness Center, in Rolling Meadows, Illinois. Non-exercisers loose
about 75 percent fat, 25 percent muscle per pound. "This may not
seem real important, but muscle affects metabolism and metabolism affects how easily we get and stay lean," she says.

This is because muscle, unlike fat, is a very active tissue. Each
pound requires 50 to 100 calories just to sustain cellular activity.
Therefore, when we sacrifice muscle to dieting, we forfeit energy
burning potential. This is why someone who once dropped ten
pounds eating 1500 calories a day without exercising may find it increasing difficult to loose weight at this rate a second time. Nega-
tively altering body composition (fat to muscle ratio) can also
require weight watchers to eat less once they have reached their diet
goal to avoid tipping the scales back to pre-diet position. Since few
of us are able to do this, "cutting calories without adding exercise
can actually make you fatter in the long run," says Wayne Westcott,
an exercise physiologist and strength training consultant to the
YMCA of U.S.A. So physical activity is essential to weight control,
"and aerobic exercise is not enough," says Westcott.

Add Weight, Loose Fat

Aerobic exercise, that which increases heart rate to between
60 and 80 percent of the maximum and maintains that rate for an
extended period of time, has long been considered the key to ballast
control. It provides a way to burn energy quickly. For example, cy-

cling and running demand up to about 600 calories an hour. It also combats what is known as the "starvation response," which is a sharp slowing of metabolic rate, or energy consumption, in reaction to restricted caloric intake. But though aerobic exercise can sometimes prevent muscle loss under dieting conditions, it cannot build muscle as efficiently as weight training. This seems to matter, according to researchers, especially as we age.

Although aerobic exercise can sometimes prevent muscle loss while dieting, it cannot build muscle as effectively as strength training. Therefore, strength training should be a part of any weight loss program.

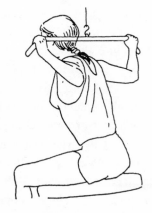

One study that reveals weight training, currently the stepsister to aerobic exercise, as the real fitness princess, compared two groups of 36 men and women after having completed an eight week program. All of them ate a reduced calorie diet made up of 20 percent fat, 20 percent protein and 60 percent carbohydrates. In addition, all participants were required to exercise three times a week, for 30 minutes a session. One group, however, combined a 15-minute total-body, strength training program with 15 minutes of aerobic exercise. The other group did 30 minutes of aerobic activities only. "The difference between the two groups was remarkable," says Westcott, the study's author. "The aerobic-exercise-only group lost an average of 3.2 pounds of fat. But the strength training/aerobic exercise group lost an average of 10 pounds of fat!" he exclaims. This group also gained two pounds of muscle each, compared to a loss of a half a pound of muscle per person among the aerobic exercisers. "There is no better way to lose fat and enhance strength and firmness," says Westcott.

A second study, conducted by researchers at Emory University in Atlanta, offers similar results. They found that overweight women who either did 20 minutes of aerobics three times a week or nothing at all, lost only 72 percent of fat per pound. "But those who did 20 minutes of circuit strength training three times a week retained more muscle," says Mary Ellen Sweeney, M.D., of the Emory Health Enhancement Program. Eighty-five percent of every pound they lost was fat. This kind of information paired with the fact that we naturally loose about a half-pound of muscle, and a resulting half-percent in metabolic rate every year from our mid-20's on, has many people rethinking their reasons for not pumping iron. The past two years have hosted a dramatic increase in the number of health clubs that offer weight machines and free weights to their clients, according to IRSA, an international trade organization for quality clubs. Professional groups, including the American College of Sports Medicine (ACSM), are also considering its worth. "Aerobic fitness needs to be the basis of any fitness routine, but to maintain musculature, you must strength train," says Michael Pollock, director of the Center for Exercise Science at the University of Florida in Gainesville. Pollock chaired the ACSM committee that put forth the revised fitness prescription just adopted by the influential organization. They now recommend that all healthy grown-ups add two strength training workouts of moderate intensity to their routines that include exercising for 20 to 60 minutes at 50 to 85 percent maximum heart rate, 3 to 5 days per week. "The evidence is overwhelming -- aerobic exercise and resistance training are equally as important to adult fitness."

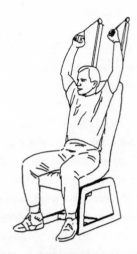

The American College of Sports Medicine has recently revised its guidelines to include at least two strength training sessions a week in addition to regular aerobic exercise.

Building Emotional Mettle

There are also a number of psychological benefits to lifting, pushing and pulling heft while reducing. For some it enhances motivation and heightens spirits. Others find they become more tuned in to their bodies and less critical of themselves both during and after weight loss.

"For me it's the mechanism that makes it all work," says Joseph Aten, 51. A recent graduate of Westcott's, he says "If I can stick to my workout schedule, I seem to have more control over what I eat." In addition, Joseph finds that monitoring his body composition, degree of strength, how he looks and feels, plus his weight frees him from the tyranny of the all-too-often fickle scale. It becomes a single means of measure rather than the sole indicator of success of failure.

For Barbara Katz, a mother of four, strength training has provided "the most incredible ego trip I've ever been on," she says. Nearly every night Barbara pops dinner into the oven and scurries down the basement stairs to leverage lead and sink into squats. "It's incredible to be 48 and feel better than you did at 28."

Judy says, "This is the first time I feel like I am doing something good for myself. Before, I was desperately trying to conform to someone else's unrealistic standards. Pounds aren't important anymore. I am working toward a healthier body. I am really proud of myself."

Francesca Gern, president of Exterior Design, Inc., a Cleveland body building clinic, says these reactions are common among the newly muscled. "When people discover what they can do to improve the bodies they have, they stop focusing on the bodies they don't have." This attitude helps people develop a total, balanced approach to fitness, rather than a fixation on weight alone. A national Gallup poll -- sponsored by American Health magazine -- shows this is a developing tendency in the general public as well. The old ideal for the ultra-thin body has become passe. Men and women are now concerned with being fit -- a goal that's both healthy and within reach for most of us. Indications of this trend are beginning to show up in the media. "Some models are meatier than they used to be," says Jeannie Ludlow Daniel, a feminist culture critic at the Center of the Study of Popular Culture in Ohio. "Women modeling swimsuits occasionally look like swimmers. This could be an indication that we are accepting different standards for different things, which could be a really good thing," she says.

Getting Started

To make sure you get all the benefits from strength training, sans frustration and injury, seek out qualified help.

"Exercise prescription in resistance training demands considerable, thorough planning, organization and evaluation," writes Steven J. Fleck, a sports physiologist in the Sports Science Program of the United States Olympic Committee. "The ability to design a successful program always requires good judgement and an under-standing of the scientific rationale for the choices made in the proc-ess," he continues. So, try to find a trainer who has a background in physical education, and experience in anatomy and biomechan-ics (credentials vary, but certification by major organizations like ACSM, the National Strength and Conditioning Association, and IDEA guarantee some degree of specialized training). Together you can assess your health and physical fitness, define specific goals and expectations, and evaluate individual needs, goals, and

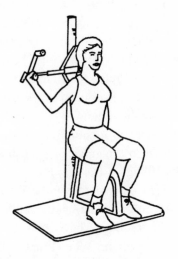

The NordicPower is a low-cost, space efficient way to work every major muscle group in the body.

demands. Then use this information to determine choice of exer-cise, order of exercise, resistance (the load used) in the exercises, length of rest between sets and exercises, and number of sets used for each exercise -- all of which are considered acute program variables. "We have found that most people realize significant change by training only every other day: 15 to 20 minutes of endurance activity (stationary cycle) and 15 to 20 minutes of strength activity (11 Nautilus machines)," says Westcott.

If you don't have time for the health club, strength training activities can also be done in the home, without complicated equipment. The new NordicPower, made by the manufacturers of NordicTrack, works out every major muscle group quickly and effectively. It's economical and compact enough to fold up and fit under the bed.

Standard Recommendations

Regardless of the program you select, there are two things that should always be included: warm-up and cool down. To effectively warm up, Westcott suggests all exercisers do five minutes of slow, rhythmic movement, such as walking, stationary cycling, running on a treadmill or calisthenics. Then stretch out the calves, thighs, back and shoulders. Do not push beyond the point of mild tension and hold your stretch for 10 to 20 seconds. To cool down simply exclude the cardiovascular work from the warmup routine. The stretches are the same.

For more information, contact local clubs and fitness centers. There are also a number of good books available: *The Nautilus Diet*, by Ellington Darden, Ph.D., and *Strength Fitness: Physiological Principles and Training Techniques,* by Wayne Westcott are both worth considering. In addition, talk to "regular" folk who do weight training. They often have valuable advice and can provide inspiration. "When I first walked in to use the machines, I felt so completely out of place," says Joseph. "Two weeks into it, I began to see results. Now I feel good about being there."

"Give it a fair shot," says Judy. "Six weeks and you'll be sold. The results are worth the discipline, but you've got to do it to believe it."

Barbell Basics

Joan Price

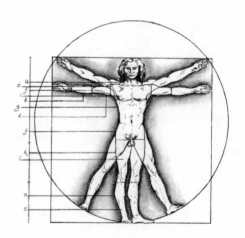

" *If you made a list of your top ten* *"*
fitness goals and never wrote the
word "muscles," this article is for
you. It is about adding some
resistance work to your exercise
routine to get the physical and
mental benefits of getting strong
and looking and feeling great.

Joan Price *is a widely published freelance writer special-*
izing in health and fitness. Her articles have appeared in
25 publications and she is working on 2 books, one for the
reluctant exerciser, the other on weight loss in collabora-
tion with The National Exercise for Life Institute. An IDEA
Foundation certified exercise instructor, Joan Price teaches
in several northern California health clubs and provides
exercise classes to San Francisco Bay Area businesses and
conventions.

11

Wait! Don't turn the page. This isn't an article for body builders or folks who envy them. In fact, if you made a list of your top ten fitness goals and never wrote the word "muscles," this article is for you. Strength training isn't about having biceps that pop your sleeves. It isn't about spending your day in the gym. It is about adding some resistance work to your exercise routine so that you get the physical and mental benefits of getting strong and looking and feeling great.

Let's sweep out the stereotypes. Women, you don't need to worry that strength training will make you look masculine. You're not going to bulk up. But you are going to develop a lean, tight, well-defined look. In fact, it can help you shape and accentuate those feminine curves. I know, you've seen the muscle men and women in magazines, and they haven't exactly sent you running out to buy a set of barbells. But keep in mind that those muscular models are competitors: they spend most of the day in rigorous training, lifting weights heavier than you'll ever attempt.

"Instead of worrying about too much muscle, the average man and woman should be concerned about too little muscle," says strength training expert Wayne Westcott, Ph.D. He explains that adults lose about one pound of muscle every two years after age 20, unless they do some form of strength training. Since most of us weigh more, not less, than we did at 20, we've replaced those lost muscle pounds with fat pounds -- and padded on some extra. Ouch.

What Does Strength Training Mean To You?

Muscle makes you look good. The super skinny look is out (thank goodness!) and the strong, shapely, toned look is in. You're already on the right track if you do aerobic exercise -- it conditions your most important muscle, the heart. Plus it burns fat and gives you energy and a rosy glow of fitness. Strength training takes up where aerobic exercise quits, helping you reshape your body and firm it up. Your new muscle awareness also helps you get more out of your aerobic workout, increasing the benefits. Strength training plus aerobic exercise are the perfect combination for balanced fitness.

Are you trying to manage your weight? The higher your metabolic rate, the faster you burn calories. That's why aerobic exercise is so important for burning fat: it not only uses stored fat as fuel after the first 20 minutes, but it raises your metabolism for hours after exercising. Strength training also raises your metabolism -- and not just for a matter of hours.

Here's why. The more muscle mass you have, the higher your metabolism, because muscle demands more calories. According to Westcott, research shows that every pound of muscle we gain raises our metabolic rate by about 50 calories a day. (Likewise, every pound of muscle we lose lowers it by the same amount.) So a person on a strength training program will burn more calories per day than a person who eats the same amount but doesn't strength train, even if they both do the same aerobic workout.

"Weight training and aerobic activity go hand in hand for changing body composition and getting results," says Jim Mobley, owner of Sunset Fitness Center in San Francisco. "Since we've added weights to our program, I've visually noticed a difference in people's bodies." The change is more than visual. When members take Sunset's fitness assessments, Mobley finds, "Inevitably, the women and men who take our weight training class always score the highest on the upper body and abdominal strength tests, and their body fat percentage tends to be within the ideal range."

Strength training helps you look and feel younger. Toned muscles fill up previously sagging skin to give your body a toned, shapely look. Your posture improves, and you feel strong and confident.

Even more important, increasing your muscle mass may be your best protection against osteoporosis. More muscle means stronger bones. This is because muscle development aids in the mineralization of bone, helping bones becomes denser. This increased density slows down the natural loss of bone mass as we get older. So don't resign yourself to getting weaker with the years -- get stronger instead.

Improved strength also helps you lead a physically active lifestyle with more energy and less risk of injury. This helps you in all parts of your life, not just your exercise hours. You'll carry kids, golf clubs and groceries without back strain, climb stairs without huffing and puffing, and pull your suitcases out of the car without wrenching your shoulder. And you'll feel powerful.

What is Strength Training?

By strength training, we mean exercise that stresses muscles to the point that they cope by getting stronger. At first, you may not even need weights or resistance other than your own body. As you get fitter, you'll find that you need more resistance -- meaning a prop that you pull, push, or lift against to make the muscle work harder.

For example, when you're first getting in shape, 15 side leg lifts may exhaust your thigh muscles. Eventually though, you're doing 15... 30... 60 with ease -- and nothing's happening. Try those leg lifts with 1- or 2-pound ankle weights and see how that changes the exercise!

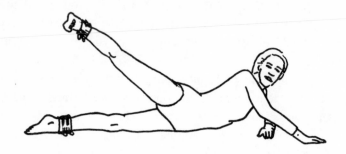

Adding weights to an exercise can greatly intensify the workout and thereby increase the benefits.

Likewise, let's say you're trying to tone that flabby under-belly of the upper arm. One way to work that area (called the triceps), is to sit up straight on a chair or bench, raise one arm up close to the head, then slowly bend at the elbow as if you're trying to touch your shoulder, keeping the upper arm and elbow close to the head. Straighten and bend a few more times, always slow and controlled. Now try the same exercise holding a light weight (1-3 pounds) in your hand. See how it intensifies the work?

Strength training is more than free weights. You can use resistance machines, available in most health clubs, where you adjust the weight on the machine, then perform the movement. For home workouts, the new Nordic Fitness Chair provides adjustable "exercise arms" with pulley cords that let you vary the resistance with the force of your movement. Those who are strong can get a substantial workout, while a deconditioned person can get a safe, challenging workout. Or you can also use exercise-weight rubber bands, surgical tubing, Dyna-Bands, or other devices that resist your movements.

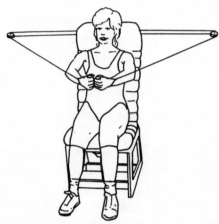

The Nordic Fitness Chair automatically varies the resistance with the force of the movement. Those who are strong can get a substantial workout, while a deconditioned person can get a safe, challenging workout.

Help! I'm Gaining Weight

Scale weight is a poor indicator of fitness. Body fat testing, a tape measure, or even photographs can give you more information than the scales about the effects of your exercise program. This is because muscle is leaner than fat, but it weighs more. So as you lose fat and gain muscle, your scale probably won't show the difference at first -- but your tape measure will.

Some people actually find that they gain weight when they start strength training because they're gaining muscle. Yet they appear slimmer and firmer, and friends remark about how lean and fit they look. Don't bury your head in the scales! Rethink your attitude, and work to change your fat/lean proportions instead of simply dropping pounds.

Staying Safe

The two keys for safety in strength training are control and technique. Control means that you perform each exercise slowly, with full attention, and without momentum. Never fling your weight or throw your whole body into the move. Be aware of which muscle you're working, and focus your awareness on the muscle. Keep the amount of weight manageable so that you can complete the move with full control.

Technique means that you understand the proper form for each exercise. If you're learning from a book or videotape, concentrate on imitating the whole body alignment, not just the limbs in motion. Look at how the back, neck and head are aligned. Are the knees bent? How much? Which body parts move? How far? How is the ending position different from the beginning? Practice without weights until you understand the form.

Tips for Effective Strength Training

1. Begin by warming up the muscles you're going to use without weights. Get the muscles and joints in motion with rhythmic movement, going through each group you plan to work. Or do ten minutes of an all-purpose exercise that warms up all you muscles for you, such as NordicTrack or striding.

2. Always perform your movements slowly. The aim isn't to get to the end of a move, but rather to feel the move every inch of the way. Return to your starting position even more slowly. Don't shorten the move or just do the part that's easy.

3. Breathe! Exhale on the lifting or pulling phase; inhale lowering or releasing. Don't hold your breath.

4. Don't overdo it. Better to do a little less than too much, especially when you're first learning your limits. Overdoing it leads to pain, discouragement, and even injury. Mild soreness the next day --a slight ache or stiffness -- is okay. It just means your muscles are adapting, and it will pass as you get stronger. But if you're feeling pain that interferes with your day, you overdid it.

5. Be careful of previous injuries. Test an injured area with no weight or ·a light weight. If there's any pain, stop. Pay particular attention to old injury sites. These areas may not be as strong as before, even though you think they're completely healed. Get medical advice about rehabilitation exercises if you find you have weak or sensitive spots.

6. Stay in tune with how your body feels at all times. If a move hurts, don't do it. Period.

7. Log your workouts. Keep track of the muscle groups worked, the amount of weight and number of repetitions ("reps") for each one. You'll be surprised at how quickly you progress.

8. Don't increase your weight until you can do 12 reps in slow, controlled, proper form. Then increase the weight or resistance slightly so that you can do only 6-8 reps.

9. Stretch each muscle group when you're done. If you don't stretch, you leave your muscles contracted, often resulting in soreness the next day and a decrease in flexibility over time. So always end your workout with five minutes of stretching.

10. For best results, strength train regularly, but no more than 2-3 times a week. Your muscles need 48 hours to recover from intense work and get stronger. Fill in those alternate days with aerobic exercise for balanced fitness.

Everyday Benefits of Strength Training

Maxine Rock

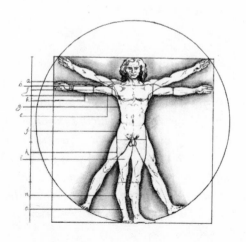

❝ *In everyday life, most of us work* **❞**
at top capacity for short periods
of time on tasks such as digging
a garden or carrying luggage.
Strength training duplicates real-
life performance with resistance
from barbells, machines, and
body weight.

Maxine Rock is a feature writer with 20 years of experi-
ence, and the author of three non-fiction books. She holds
14 awards for excellence in writing, including the 1988
Gold Award first place prize in Medical Journalism for na-
tional magazine writing about health. She is the Special
Assignment Editor and medical columnist for BUSINESS
ATLANTA and founder and editor of THE HEALTH
LETTER, a quarterly on health and medicine. Her per-
sonal interests included fitness training, running, and
cross-country skiing.

12

I can lug the laundry down to the basement now, easily lifting a basket filled with soggy towels and yesterday's sweat-soaked jogging pants.

Opening stubborn jar lids is a snap.

It's no longer necessary for me to wait until an overworked teenager shows up to load the groceries into my car, and I could even start the lawnmower -- and push it around the blanket of weeds we call grass -- if the yard man doesn't show up.

These everyday tasks haven't gotten easier. It's just that I am stronger now because of a balanced fitness training program. Instead of concentrating just on aerobics, which has kept me slim and fit, I'm using my upper body muscles too. The result has been a burst of strength I didn't know was possible for a 49-year-old woman. It's changed the way I think about the whole concept of "fitness."

For a long time, I've been devoting at least four sessions a week to huff-and-puff cardiovascular exercises such as running, aerobic dancing, or using a machine that simulates cross-country skiing. These exercises have helped keep my heart healthy and contributed to lower blood pressure and cholesterol counts. But I never did strength training exercises for the muscles in my upper body, because it never dawned on me that the effort might be worthwhile. Besides, who wants bulging biceps? What would I do with extra strength if I had it?

Plenty, it's turned out. It was my aerobics instructor who convinced me to give strength training a try, and in the year since I began I've noticed an immense difference in my body -- and in the ease with which I conduct my daily life. It's not just prowess in lugging laundry and lifting groceries that's at stake here. It's fending off the ravages of advancing age and keeping an erect, youthful body.

"As you get older, your body will slump if you're not in good shape through strength training," says Atlanta fitness expert Tony deLeede. "That's one reason why some older women look bent. Their stomach muscles and shoulder muscles literally can't hold them up. A person who's been strength training is better able to stand erect, and usually doesn't have those age-related pot bellies or flabby arms and chest muscles. Women don't have to worry about getting muscular, because bulging muscles don't develop without a great deal of time and effort. . . if they develop in a woman at all." .

Even though I've been thin (and definitely not muscle-bound) for most of my adult life because I'm so active, I did notice poor posture and the beginning of a pop-out stomach as middle age came nearer. I tried to head off the trouble with more exercise, but it seemed that no amount of running or aerobic dancing did the trick. Finally, I asked some other women how they kept that firm, well-shaped look. Their answer? Strength training.

"A carefully controlled program of weight resistance exercises shapes your body," says Sara Mack Lawson, a 42-year-old exercise physiologist. "As you start aging, that is particularly important as a way to stay attractive and strong. Also, strength training does help in weight control. The way to keep your metabolism higher is to have a larger percentage of muscle than body fat. You can do that through strength training."

A carefully planned program of an aerobic activity such as cross-country skiing with strength training will greatly improve the quality of your life.

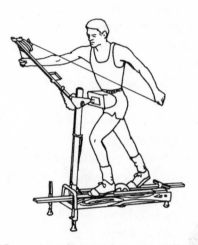

After the age of about 35, a person's muscle mass shrinks three to six percent every decade... unless he or she stays active and constantly uses those muscles. In everyday life, most of us work at top capacity for short periods of time on tasks such as digging a garden or carrying luggage. Then we rest, and tackle the job again. Strength training duplicates real-life performance with resistance from barbells, machines, large exercise rubber bands, body weight or devices such as the convenient new Nordic Fitness Chair by Nordic Track. This unique device utilizes an isokinetic resistance mechanism that provides a complete upper body workout in as little as 10 minutes. Its attractive design makes it appropriate for use right in the living area of the home.

Some experts use the term "isotonics" for the usual strength training movements of lifting or pulling an object to a predetermined level, then returning it to its original position. Others prefer "isokinetics" which is working against resistance that accommodates itself to the force you put into the movement. For example, an isotonic machine will allow you to set it for ten pounds of force.

You get that same ten pounds through the entire movement. An isokinetic machine, such as the Nordic Fitness Chair, will give you ten pounds of resistance if you pull slowly, but a lot more than that if you pull fast. It's a more flexible machine because it provides resistance depending on the force you exert as your body completes an entire range of motion.

No matter what you use -- weights, machines, or the laundry basket -- adding strength training to your exercise routine provides what I now refer to as "balanced fitness." While aerobics will always be the foundation of my exercise routine, here are the extra benefits that I'm reaping from spending time on strength training, too:

- Reduced susceptibility to injury, because of stronger muscles and tendons
- Greater flexibility
- Improved coordination and body movement
- Improved appearance
- Better posture
- An end to backaches
- Some protection against osteoporosis

When I look back on the days when I did only aerobics, it seems that I spent a lot of time and energy on just the lower half of my body. Other people tell me they have the same sensation about short-changing the upper half of their bodies until they tried strength training.

"I feel and look a lot different since I added strength training," says 29-year-old Pam Thompson. "My buttocks are much firmer, and I got rid of flabby arms. Also, I know it has helped me in everyday life. The other day I was working in the yard with my husband, making flower beds, and he was delighted when I could lift big rocks off the truck by myself!"

Pam lifts 70 pounds on the bench press in two sets of ten times each, and works against 85 pound leg weights in two sets of eight

Strength training provides a constant challenge that can prevent boredom with an exercise routine.

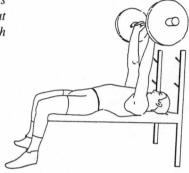

times each. Gail deLeede, 37 works with slightly heavier weights three times a week and says she noticed new "muscle definition" and "a slimmer, trimmer body" in just eight weeks. She also credits strength training with giving her the extra power she needs to lift her 20-pound baby in one arm, and juggle a bag of groceries in the other. "I really feel good about being able to do that," she says, "and being able to press 75 pounds when I could only do 65 pounds last week. Strength training is a constant challenge."

After ten years of doing the same old exercises, the "constant challenge" provided by weight training gives me the extra zing I need to keep from becoming bored with fitness. I can reach a certain goal and stay there, or I can make things more interesting by setting a new goal. Sometimes I just trade in my hand-held weights for a heavier set, and sometimes I merely adjust the pressure of the weight machine. I stay away from gadgets that require making complicated adjustments; it's no fun to fiddle with those contraptions when you have a limited amount of time to spend on fitness.

For now, adding an extra 30 minutes of strength training to my aerobics workout three or four times a week does the trick. Maybe later -- when I'm retired -- I'll be ready for a greater challenge. In the meantime, thanks to strength training, laundry baskets and lawnmowers are a cinch.